Electrocardiography of Acute Myocardial Ischaemic Syndromes

Electrocardiography of Acute Myocardial Ischaemic Syndromes

Edited by

Samuel Sclarovsky, MD
Head of Department of Cardiology
Rabin Medical Center (Beilinson Campus) and
Professor of Cardiology
Sackler School of Medicine
Tel Aviv University
Tel Aviv
Israel

MARTIN DUNITZ

© Martin Dunitz Ltd 1999

First published in the UK in 1999 by
Martin Dunitz Ltd
The Livery House
7–9 Pratt Street
London NW1 0AE

A CIP catologue record for this book is available from the British Library.

ISBN 1-85317-380-0

Distributed in the United States by:
Blackwell Science Inc
Commerce Place, 350 Main Street
Malden MA 02148
USA
Tel: +1 800 215 1000

Distributed in Canada by:
Login Brothers Book Company
324 Salteaux Crescent
Winnipeg MB R3J 3T2
Canada
Tel: +1 204 224 4068

Distributed in Brazil by:
Ernesto Reichmann Distribuidora de Livros, Ltda
Rua Coronel Marques 335
Tatuape 03440-000
São Paolo
Brazil

Composition by Wearset, Boldon, Tyne and Wear
Printed and bound in Spain

In memory of my unforgettable parents
Paulina and Jacobo

To my beloved wife *Esther (Kuky)*
and our daughters
Daniela, Fabiana and Sharon

To *Maurico B Rosenbaum* MD
The 'master' that taught me the power of clinical electrocardiography

To *Professor Jacob Agmon*
The 'director' that believed in me and my work

'My teachers gave me knowledge, but they were surpassed by my students' (Talmud)

Professor Abraham Caspi MD, Professor Boris Strasberg MD, Reuben Levin MD,
Alex Arditti MD, Oscar Kracoff MD, Nili Zafrir MD, Alik Sagie MD, Eldad Rechavia MD,
Haim Kusniec MD, Aviv Mager MD, Yochai Birnbaum MD, David Hasdai MD,
Tuvia Ben-Gal MD, Abed Assali MD and Bruria Zlotikamien MD

Contents

Acknowledgements

I would like to acknowledge my secretary, Mrs Judith Har-Kedar, for her support and her important contribution towards the publication of this book.

To Galen S Wagner MD for his wise advice in the early stages of writing this book, and to David Hasdai MD for his great assistance in the preparation of the final manuscript which made it possible to accomplish this publication.

I would also like to thank my publishers Martin Dunitz Ltd, and in particular, Yasmin Khan-Chowdhury and Alan Burgess, for their invaluable help in getting this book to press.

Preface

An editorial in a recent publication in Paris emphasized that since the late 1960s to the present day conventional surface electrocardiography has been somewhat neglected, as priority has been given to invasive electrophysiology. In apparent contradiction to the above, the number of books written on this subject during this period has been immense. With the exception of a modest number of books, such as Rosenbaum and Sodi Pallares, those published in English have not been innovative. The future of clinical electrocardiology could reside in the electrocardiogram (if used properly; preferably with the assistance of the latest computer technology).

Samuel Sclarovsky offers us this masterpiece, which for proper evaluation requires an understanding of the author's psychodynamics. Beyond any doubt, he is a talented, renaissance man, not only a person with an inborn endowment, but practically a genius since he fulfills the necessary integration of original scientific, sociological, metaphysical and psychological factors to be considered as such. Samuel Sclarovsky is in a sense, a man 'possessed', who for many years has been, against overwhelming odds, totally and completely immersed in (or, rather obsessed with) the subject. This quasi-compulsive intuitive and acquired experience has provided the material for this book.

The book includes non-conventional, original, novel knowledge (about which we do not know as much as we think) providing easy as well as, what at first glance appears, difficult aspects of the topic. Consequently, to be fully understood, one must begin to read it with an *a-priori* premise which requires the abandonment of conventional ways of thinking while being prepared to proceed in different directions.

The author has written about the electrocardiography of what can be, in a general way, considered as acute ischaemic processes (including myocardial infarction) using experience accumulated over three decades by spending long hours at the patient's side. This *sui-generis* approach merits serious consideration.

I suggest that the reader read in the proper order (not proceeding directly to a chapter where a topic of interest may reside) but to rather concentrate, understand, and (if possible, at the beginning) memorize the phases of the ischaemic processes as defined and properly explained in Chapter 1.

Finally, the publisher, Martin Dunitz Ltd, should be congratulated for making the book available. They understood its uniqueness amongst the vast ocean of other books, going beyond to the part of the text stating after ('vanity of vanities, all is vanity') that 'there is nothing new under the sun'. On the contrary, they understood what the author must have said at the beginning of his enterprise, namely, 'but I gave my heart to seek and search, out of wisdom, things that are under heaven.'

Agustin Castellanos
Professor of Medicine
Jackson Memorial Hospital
University of Miami
Florida, USA

Introduction

At the beginning of 1960, I had the unique opportunity of joining the cardiology training program at the Ramos Mejía Hospital in Buenos Aires, Argentina. I was assigned to the group headed by Mauricio Rosenbaum, one of this century's most prominent electrocardiographists. Through his teachings, I became fascinated with the wealth of information that could be derived from a simple ECG tracing. At that time, more sophisticated diagnostic devices were not yet available, and the ECG thus became a valuable tool to the practising cardiologist.

In the early 1960s most of the data that was available about the diagnostic significance of the ECG pertained to congenital and valvular diseases. There were few data regarding the ECG manifestations of ischaemic heart disease. It was only in the early 1970s that the field of electrocardiography in ischaemic heart disease began to flourish, concomitantly with the advent of new devices that enabled the diagnosis of coronary artery disease.

Being a physician attending to patients in the coronary intensive care unit, I was fascinated by the ability of the ECG to diagnose acute ischaemic episodes accurately and to predict outcome. Over more than 30 years, I have dedicated my research endeavours to the investigation of unique ECG patterns in ischaemic heart disease. These efforts have attempted to correlate ECG findings with other imaging modalities such as coronary angiography, echocardiography, and nuclear medicine. This book summarizes the current knowledge concerning the ECG in ischaemic heart disease, reflecting my previous reports as well as those of others.

Chapter 1 Angina at rest and acute myocardial ischaemia

SUMMARY

The electrocardiogram (ECG) recorded during the acute ischaemia of angina at rest, as well as during the ensuing recovery phases, is of diagnostic, therapeutic, and prognostic significance. Serial ECG recordings offer unique insight into the underlying mechanisms of the ischaemic process. The ischaemic process can be divided into three ECG phases.

PHASE I

Evidence of a sudden imbalance between demand and supply of oxygen to the myocardium. The ECGs obtained during this phase are characterized by two main patterns.

Pattern 1, regional ischaemia is characterized by the appearance of new peaked and tall T waves. Pattern 2 is characterized by transient ST segment depression in precordial leads with inverted T waves, reflecting an acute increase in the left ventricular end diastolic pressure (LVEDP) that is caused by circumferential subendocardial ischaemia.

PHASE II

This phase of the ischaemic process reflects the restoration of the supply–demand balance. The changes that occur during this phase are determined by the type of changes that occurred during the first phase of the ischaemic process.

PHASE III

This phase encompasses the ECG changes that occur several days after the acute ischaemic event. These changes relate only to regional myocardial ischaemia and entail four different scenarios in the configuration of the T waves:

- progressive normalization of the T wave from inverted to upright;
- pseudonormalization during a recurring ischaemic event, manifested by an acutely upright T wave that was previously inverted;
- persistently upright T waves; and
- persistently negative T waves.

Identifying these patterns is of therapeutic and prognostic significance.

INTRODUCTION

Angina at rest is a subtype of unstable angina. It portends a high risk of subsequent morbidity and mortality.[1] The ECG recorded during the acute episode is critical for the diagnosis.[2] The ECG is an objective reflection of the series of events that occur in the myocardium during the acute ischaemic syndrome, for it demonstrates the metabolic, electrophysiological and haemodynamic consequences of the acute ischaemia. Moreover, the ECG can demonstrate these parameters even during asymptomatic ischaemic episodes (silent ischaemia).[3]

The ECG manifestations of acute ischaemia can be divided into three phases (*Fig. 1.1*).

PHASE I OF ACUTE ISCHAEMIA

Phase I of acute ischaemia as manifested in the ECG occurs when there is evidence of a sudden imbalance between demand and supply of oxygen to the myocardium. The ECGs obtained during this phase are characterized by two main patterns.

PATTERN 1

Pattern 1, regional ischaemia, is characterized by the appearance of new peaked and tall T waves (*Fig. 1.2*). These T waves are caused by the sudden

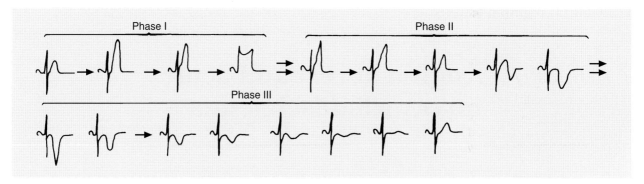

Figure 1.1 *A depiction of the ECG patterns in the evolution of acute myocardial ischaemia. Three serial ECG phases may be noted with different patterns in each phase. The first four ECG complexes illustrate the ECG patterns in Phase I, reflecting the sudden reduction in coronary blood flow in an epicardial artery. The next five complexes demonstrate the ECG patterns in Phase II, reflecting the restoration of the coronary blood flow (reperfusion). The serial ECG changes are reciprocal to those in Phase 1. The last eight complexes show the late ECG changes occurring in Phase III, with gradual return to baseline.*

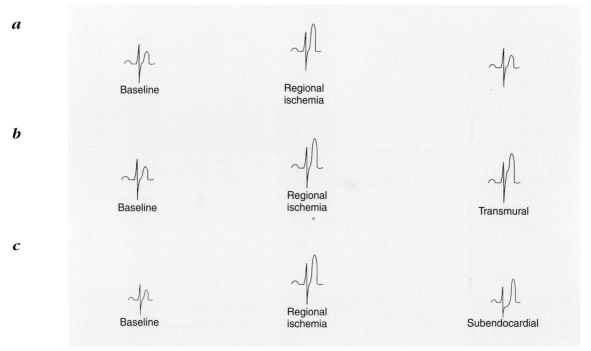

Figure 1.2 *(a) The first complex was obtained at baseline. The second complex depicts a tall, peaked T wave, reflecting regional ischaemia. The third beat demonstrates the return to baseline after resolution of ischaemia. (b) The first complex was obtained at baseline. The second complex again demonstrates regional ischaemia, as explained in (a). The third complex depicts the development of transmural ischaemia, characterized by ST-segment elevation and tall, peaked T waves. (c) The regional ischaemia eventually culminates in subendocardial ischaemia (third complex), characterized by ST-segment depression and tall, peaked T waves.*

and transient narrowing or obstruction (either complete or incomplete) of an epicardial artery.[4] These ECG changes are usually confined to the region of the heart supplied by one epicardial artery. The ischaemic area is usually surrounded by healthy myocardium. Thus, this pattern delineates regional ischaemia. The changes in the configuration of the T waves stem from the metabolic and electrophysiological changes occurring in the area of ischaemia.[5]

Transmural regional ischaemia

Transmural regional ischaemia is a subtype of regional ischaemia. It is characterized by:

- transient ECG changes;
- peaked and tall T waves;
- ST segment elevation; and
- the absence of tachycardia (heart rate <90 beats per minute) (see *Fig. 1.2b*).

The first change that occurs in transmural regional ischaemia is the development of peaked and tall T waves. If the ischaemic process is enhanced, ST segment elevation may be evident, and this is possibly followed by an alteration of the terminal portion of the QRS complex (*Fig. 1.3*). Because these succes-sive ECG changes are related to the intensity of the ischaemia, it is possible to grade the process (*Fig. 1.4*):

- Ischaemia Grade 1: peaked and tall T waves;
- Ischaemia Grade 2: appearance of ST segment elevation;
- Ischaemia Grade 3: distortion of the terminal vector of the QRS complex.

Transmural regional ischaemia is caused by an acute and complete obstruction of a coronary artery. The obstruction can be either mechanical, as in a thrombus, or 'functional', as in vasoconstriction[6] or collapse.[7] The series of ECG changes progress from one grade of ischaemia to the next (*Fig. 1.5*). This phenomenon can be also demonstrated in the

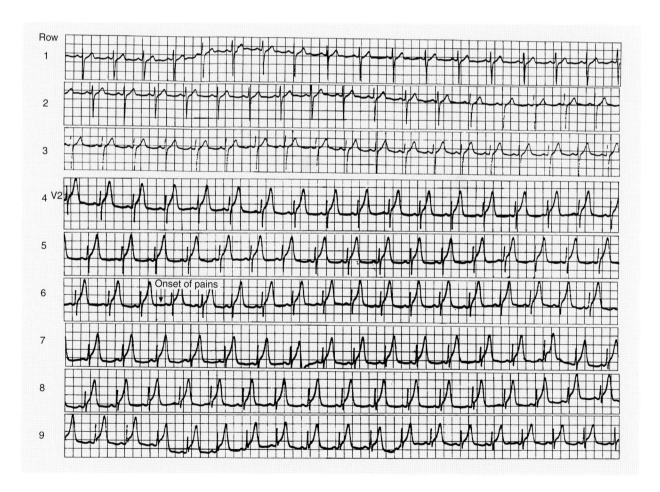

Figure 1.3 *Continuous ECG recordings from lead V2. Characteristic ECG patterns in the evolution of regional transmural ischaemia. In the first complexes, the T wave becomes progressively more prominent in amplitude until the end of the third row. In rows 4–7, the ST segment gradually rises. In row 8, the S wave diminishes until its disappearance in the middle of row 9.*

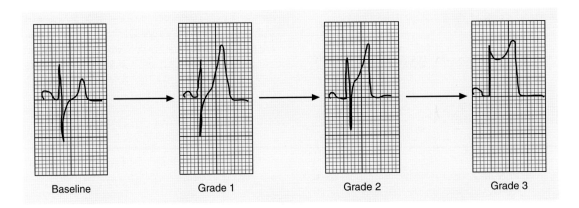

Figure 1.4 *The different ECG grades of ischaemia during regional transmural ischaemia.*

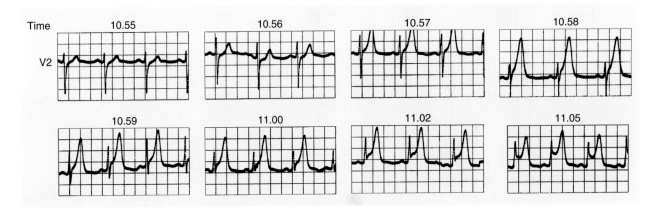

Figure 1.5 *Ten minutes of continuous ECG recording in lead V2 in a patient with regional transmural ischaemia. The T wave becomes more prominent over time until 10.57 (ischaemia Grade 1). Thereafter, the ST segment begins to rise (Grade 2). At 10.59, the terminal portion of the QRS complex becomes distorted, with the disappearance of the S wave and an increase in the amplitude of the R wave (Grade 3).*

catheterization laboratory when the coronary artery is occluded by a balloon catheter (*Fig. 1.6*), and in animals in the experimental laboratory (*Fig. 1.7*).

In some patients the ischaemic process is arrested at Grade 2 and does not progress to Grade 3. These patients develop only ischaemia Grade 2 during an acute ischaemic transmural regional event (*Fig. 1.8*). This probably reflects a protective mechanism that has been developed by the myocardium. Indeed, other patients may even develop only Grade 1 ischaemia without further progression (*Fig. 1.9*). The myocardium may be protected by two mechanisms: collateral circulation or preconditioning of the myocardium.[8,9] Patients who develop only Grade 1 are more likely to be protected by collateral circula-

tion, whereas patients who develop Grade 2 are more likely to be protected by preconditioning of the myocardium.

Obstruction of the left anterior descending artery during coronary angioplasty causes different ECG patterns. The author performed continuous 12-channel ECG recordings during coronary angioplasty in order to evaluate better the effect of the obstruction on the myocardium. In all cases, there was no previous myocardial pathology, there was obstruction of more than 75% of the left anterior descending artery, there was no collateral circulation, and the obstruction was below the first diagonal artery. At least three inflations of the balloon no less than 2 minutes apart were performed.

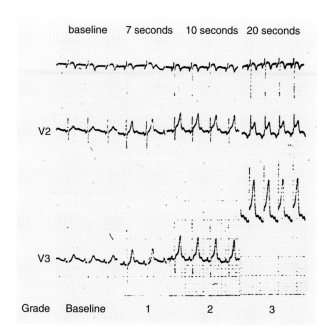

Figure 1.6 *The evolution of the three ECG grades of ischaemia in leads V2 and V3 during balloon inflation in the proximal left anterior descending coronary artery. Note the progression from Grade 1 to 2 and then to Grade 3. These changes occurred over 20 seconds.*

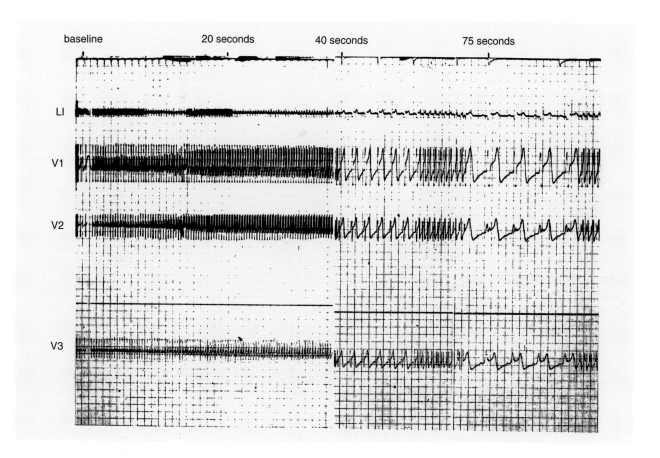

Figure 1.7 *Balloon inflation in the left anterior descending artery in an experimental canine model. There is a progression from Grade 1 to Grade 3 through Grade 2. These changes occurred over 75 seconds after occlusion of the artery by the balloon.*

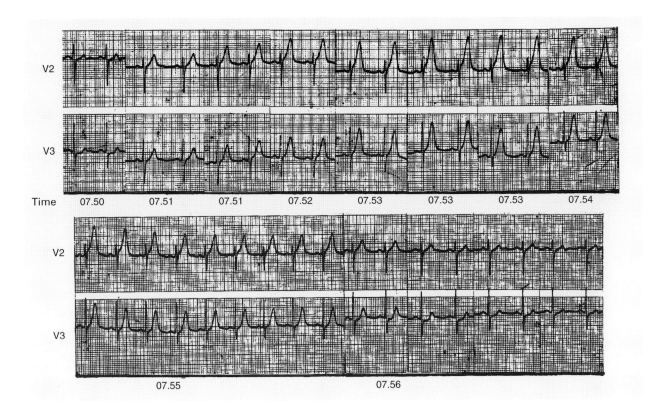

Figure 1.8 *Continuous ECG monitoring during regional transmural ischaemia. The T waves became more prominent in leads V2 and V3 with mild ST segment elevation. However, the ECG pattern does not progress to Grade 3. At 07.56, the ECG shows gradual recovery (Phase II).*

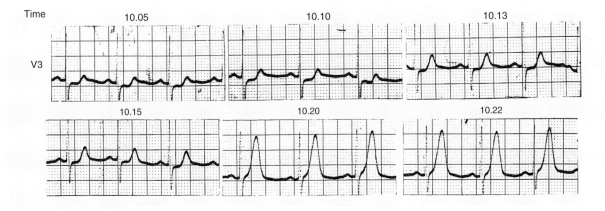

Figure 1.9 *Continuous ECG recordings over 17 minutes of ischaemia. The patient developed prominent T waves, but never progressed beyond Grade 1 of ischaemia.*

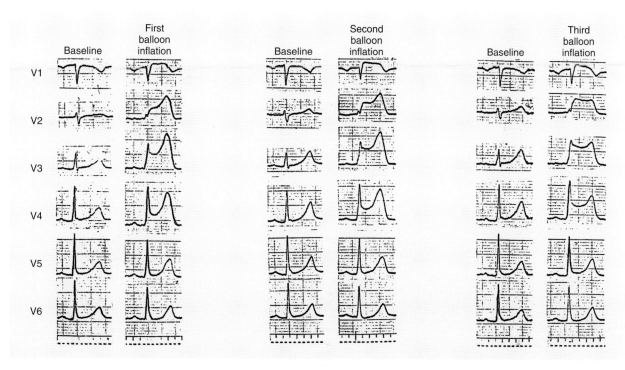

Figure 1.10   *ECG recordings during angioplasty during three balloon inflations and the preceding baselines. The patient developed the same ECG pattern of ischaemia Grade 3 during each one of the three balloon inflations.*

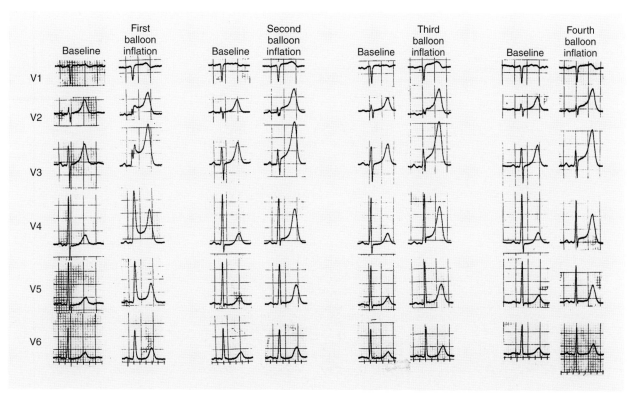

Figure 1.11   *ECG recordings during angioplasty during four balloon inflations and the preceding baselines. During the first balloon inflation, the patient developed ischaemia Grade 3. During the second and third inflations, the patient developed ischaemia Grade 2. During the last balloon inflation, only Grade 1 ischaemia was evident.*

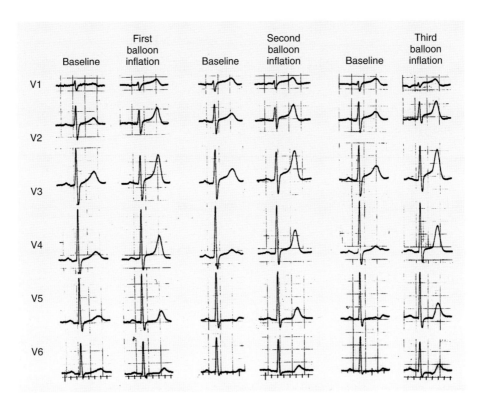

Figure 1.12 *ECG recordings during angioplasty during three balloon inflations and the preceding baselines. The patient developed only Grade 2 ischaemia during each of the three inflations.*

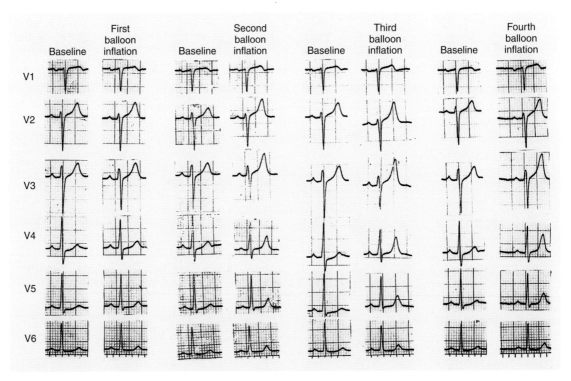

Figure 1.13 *ECG recordings during angioplasty during four balloon inflations and the preceding baselines. Note that the patient never developed ST segment elevation during the balloon inflations. However, the T waves became more prominent, reflecting ischaemia Grade 1.*

Four types of ECG patterns were obtained in these experiments:

(a) Evolution to Grade 3 during all obstructions (*Fig. 1.10*). This may reflect an unprotected myocardium.

(b) Evolution to Grade 3 during the first inflation of the balloon, and Grade 2 or Grade 1 in the next inflations (*Fig. 1.11*). This may reflect the development of a protective mechanism by the myocardium.

(c) Evolution to Grade 2 during all inflations of the balloon (*Fig. 1.12*). This may reflect a partially protected myocardium.

(d) Evolution to Grade 1 in all inflations of the balloon (*Fig. 1.13*). This may reflect a well-protected myocardium.

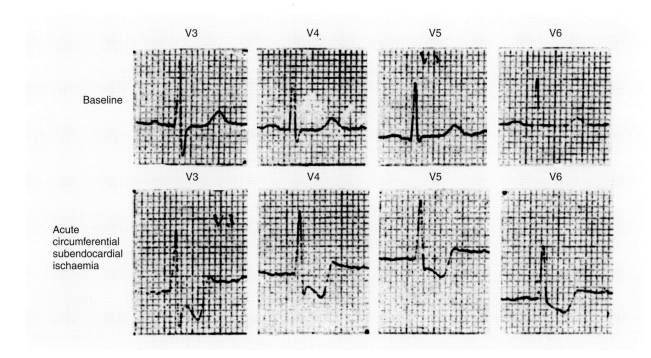

Figure 1.14 *Baseline ECG and ECG during acute circumferential subendocardial ischaemia, which is characterized by precordial ST segment depression with inverted T waves in the leads with the greatest R wave amplitude (leads V4 and V5). Note the absence of tachycardia.*

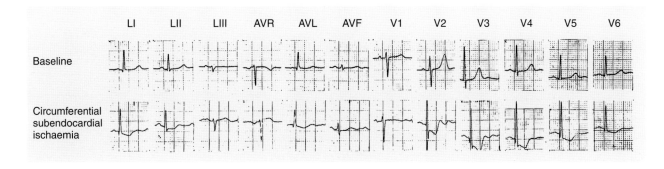

Figure 1.15 *ECG tracings at baseline and during circumferential subendocardial ischaemia, which is characterized by ST segment depression in precordial leads during pain and inverted T waves. Note the absence of tachycardia (heart rate of 60 beats per minute).*

PATTERN 2

Pattern 2 is characterized by transient ST segment depression in precordial leads, with inverted T waves. These changes are maximal in leads V4 and V5 (*Fig. 1.14*). This pattern can be further divided based on the concomitant absence (*Fig. 1.15*) or presence (*Fig. 1.16*) of tachycardia.[10] When it is not associated with tachycardia it usually reflects an acute reduction in coronary flow;[11] when it is associated with tachycardia, it is a more benign condition that reflects an acute increase in myocardial demand (see *Fig. 1.16*).

Pattern 2 reflects an acute increase in the LVEDP. This increase is due to circumferential subendocardial ischaemia, and it can, in turn, further exacerbate the ischaemic process by increasing the tension on the myocardium and decreasing blood flow.[12] The ECG changes in Pattern 2 (without concomitant tachycardia) are often the result of extensive myocardial ischaemia caused by an acute obstruction of the left main coronary artery or its equivalents, or by severe triple-vessel coronary artery disease (*Figs 1.17, 1.18*).

The advanced grades of circumferential ischaemias produce almost life-threatening effects with acute severe oedema.[13] However, in some cases of slow progression, three grades can be evaluated (*Fig. 1.19*):

- Ischaemia Grade 1: depression of the ST segment and inverted T waves;
- Ischaemia Grade 2: depressed ST segment and markedly inverted T waves, or the appearance of S waves in leads V4 and V5;
- Ischaemia Grade 3: further deepening of the inverted T wave and the S waves.

It is important to distinguish those patients with ST segment depression due to circumferential ischaemia from those who have ST segment depression due to other causes, such as hypertrophic cardiomyopathy, aortic stenosis, or chronic hypertension. Moreover, those patients with other diseases may develop ischaemia, and this must be detected; during the acute ischaemic event, ST segment depression becomes marked in leads V4 and V5 with negative T waves (*Fig. 1.20*). It seems that in such cases there is diffuse coronary artery disease or disease of the left main coronary artery. When the ST segments are less depressed and the T waves less negative, it is likely that there is a single lesion with moderate LVEDP elevation (*Fig. 1.21*).

The greatest ST segment depression is always seen in the precordial lead with the highest R wave. This is usually lead V4 or V5. When there is counter-clockwise rotation, the maximal depression in circumferential ischaemias appears in leads V3 and V4 (*Fig. 1.22*). When there is clockwise rotation of the heart, the maximal depression appears in leads V5 and V6 (*Fig. 1.23*).

The ECG characteristics of tachycardia-induced circumferential ischaemia are:

- precordial ST-segment depression (maximal in leads V4 and V5) with inverted T waves (see *Fig. 1.31*), and
- a heart rate more than 90 beats per minute.[11]

The clinical characteristics are:

- the pain may last a long time; and
- rarely is there evolution to an infarction.

When the heart rate decreases, the pain disappears and the ST segment returns to the isoelectric line.

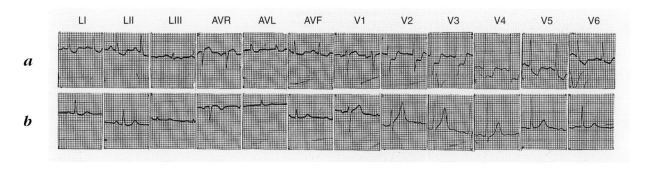

Figure 1.16 *(a) Circumferential subendocardial ischaemia during tachycardia (110 beats per minute) in a patient with single-artery coronary artery disease. (b) The patient had ST segment depression in precordial leads with inverted T waves (maximal in leads V4 and V5). These changes disappeared when normal heart rate was restored.*

a

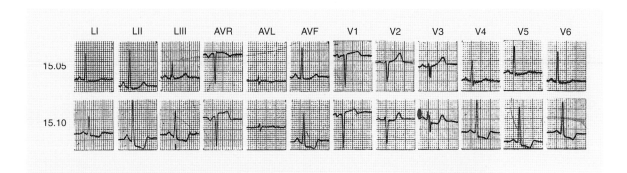

b

c

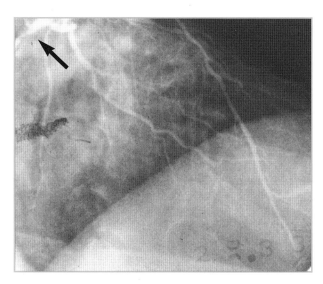

Figure 1.17   *(a) ECG tracings from a patient with acute circumferential subendocardial ischaemia. (b) Thalluim scintigraphy; during the acute episode thallium was injected, depicting uptake in the lungs (left panels, see arrows) without filling defects. Subsequent images illustrated that uptake was no longer evident, concomitantly with the resolution of the ECG changes (right panels). (c) Severe stenosis of the left main coronary artery (arrow) was detected during coronary angiography.*

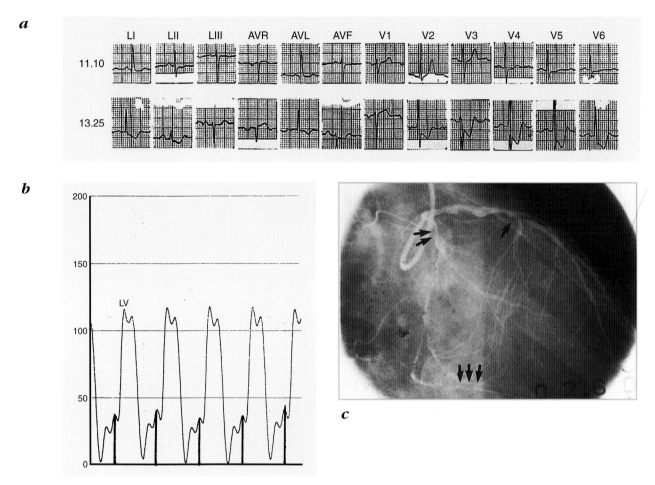

Figure 1.18 *(a) The upper row depicts the baseline tracing. In the bottom row there was ST-segment depression maximally in lead V4 through V6. This tracing was obtained during severe angina. (b) During the acute ischaemia, the patient had increased left ventricular end-diastolic pressure (LVEDP). An LVEDP of 37 mmHg denotes increased filling pressure, resulting in increased tension on the myocardium. (c) Coronary angiography performed thereafter revealed severe narrowing of all three major epicardial arteries. The lone arrow highlights a severe stenosis of the left anterior descending coronary artery, whereas the double arrows point to a stenosis in the left circumflex. The triple arrows denote collateral circulation to the right posterior descending coronary artery, indicating severe disease also in the right coronary artery.*

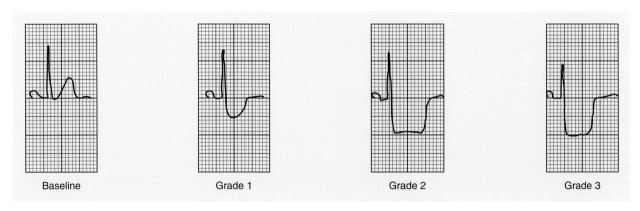

Figure 1.19 *Different ECG grades of ischaemia during circumferential subendocardial ischaemia.*

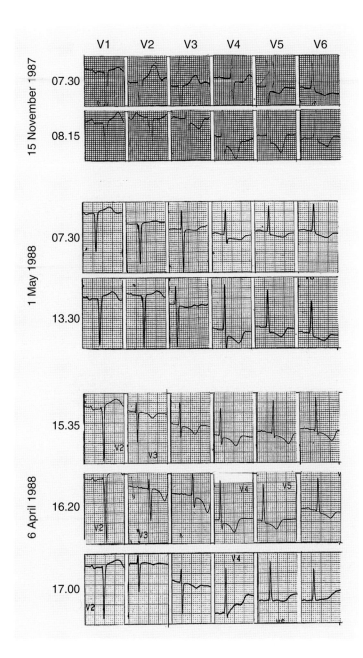

Figure 1.20 *ECG tracings from a patient with left ventricular hypertrophy attributed to chronic hypertension. The patient had chronic ST segment depression. However, during acute ischaemia not related to tachycardia, the ST segment depression became more prominent as did the T wave inversion. This patient also had severe coronary artery disease.*

This type of ischaemia is commonly caused by the pro-ischaemic effect of anti-anginal drugs such as nitrates or nifedipine, which also cause reflex tachycardia. Regardless of its aetiology, tachycardia produces a sudden increase in the LVEDP without a corresponding increase in the diastolic volume.[14]

Tachycardia has two other significant characteristics: it reduces diastolic time, the phase in which the subendocardial circulation is supplied;[15] and the epicardial circulation is not affected. It also produces a 'steal syndrome' from the left ventricular coronary flow towards the right ventricle.[16]

The circumferential type of ischaemia differs from subendocardial regional ischaemia, which is characterized by ST segment depression with upright T waves, usually in leads V3 and V4.[17] The cause of this type of ischaemia is generally a subtotal obstruction of the left anterior descending artery or a total obstruction of the first diagonal or intermediate artery (see *Fig. 1.2b*). As with the changes described above for regional transmural ischaemia, there is a cascade of ECG changes in this form of ischaemia. The first change is the appearance of positive and tall T waves. The second change is the appearance

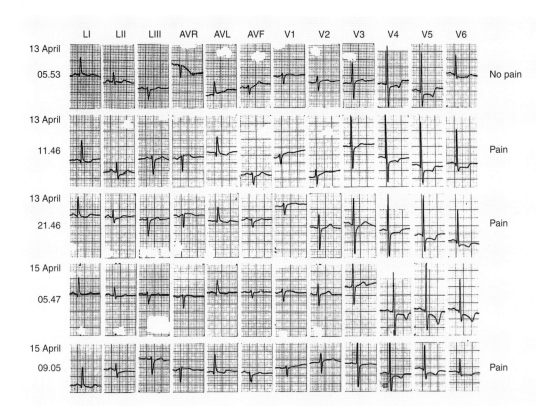

Figure 1.21 *ECG tracings from a patient with left ventricular hypertrophy due to severe aortic stenosis. During pain, the ST segment is less depressed, and the T wave becomes more upright. This patient had coronary artery disease confined to the circumflex artery.*

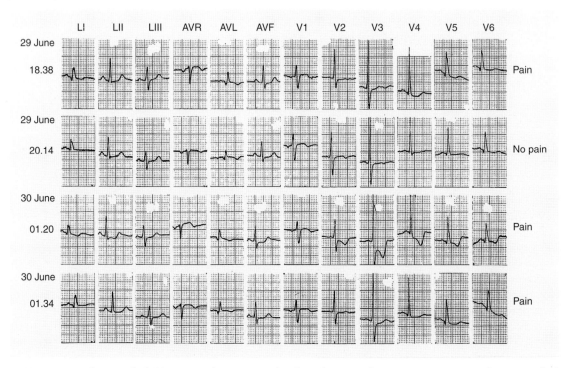

Figure 1.22 *Maximal precordial ST segment depression in lead V3 during ischaemia in a patient with counterclockwise rotation.*

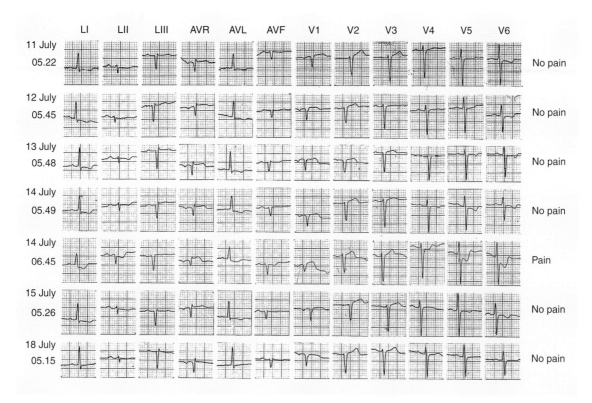

Figure 1.23   *Maximal precordial ST segment depression in leads V5 and V6 during ischaemia in a patient with clockwise rotation.*

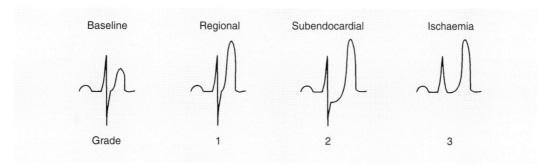

Figure 1.24   *ECG grades of ischaemia during regional subendocardial ischaemia.*

of ST segment depression. The third change is the alteration of the terminal portion of the QRS complex.

The ECG cascade in subendocardial regional ischaemias reveals the process of the ischaemic cascade in the affected area (*Fig. 1.24*).

Ischaemia Grade 1

This is manifest in the ECG by peaked and tall T waves, caused by hyperpolarization of the epicardial layer.

Ischaemia Grade 2

This is manifest in the ECG by ST segment depression, caused by the creation of an injury vector oriented from the epicardial area to the subendocardium.[18] In order for this phenomenon to occur, the lesion has to be severe, with a marked decrease in pH in the subendocardium.[19] The epicardial area might be more protected than the subendocardial area either because of subtotal acute obstruction of the left anterior descending artery or because the epicardial layer is preconditioned in relation to the subendocardium. The oxygen consumption of the subendocardial layer is 20% higher than that of the epicardial area and therefore the subendocardial layer is more affected.

Ischaemia Grade 3

This is manifest in the ECG by an alteration in the terminal portion of the QRS complex.[20] This could be the result of severe depression of conduction velocity in the Purkinje system, with late depolarization developing. The alteration of the terminal portion of QRS complex is independent of the orientation of the ST segment.

Recurrent episodes of subendocardial regional ischaemia may appear with different grades of ischaemia (*Figs 1.25, 1.26*). Alternatively, they sometimes evolve to infarction, with a unique morphology (*Fig. 1.27*). Some cases of subendocardial regional ischaemia evolve to transmural ischaemia, perhaps because of the progression from acute and incomplete occlusion to complete occlusion (*Fig. 1.28*).

Because of the clinical and prognostic importance of the acute, non-tachycardia ischaemias that cause ST segment depression and negative T waves, it is important to differentiate them from other ischaemias that cause ST segment depression in the anterior leads. ST segment depression in leads V1–V3 is commonly related to posterior ischaemia.[21] In these cases, ST segment elevation and positive T waves are also seen in leads V7 and V8. The diagnosis is very

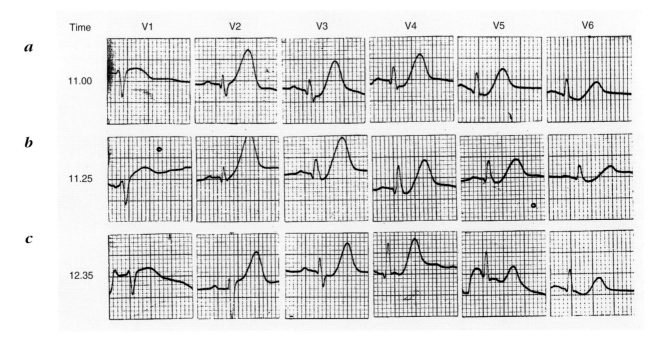

Figure 1.25 *(a) ST segment depression with upright T waves in a patient with regional subendocardial ischaemia (Grade 2). (b) Twenty-five minutes later, the S wave disappears, denoting Grade 3, but at 12:35 (c) Grade 2 ischaemia was evident again.*

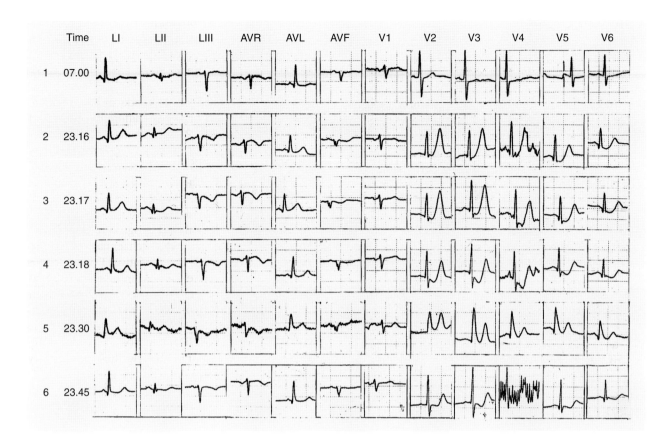

Figure 1.26 *At baseline (top row), there are minor deformities in the ST–T complex. The second and third rows illustrate regional subendocardial ischaemia Grade 3. Note the tall and peaked T waves and the slight ST segment depression in leads V2–V4. Row 4 demonstrates ischaemia Grade 2, characterized by the reappearance of the S wave with ST segment depression and upright T waves. The bottom row depicts ischaemia Grade 1.*

important when depression in leads V1 and V3 is the only sign of ischaemia in a 12-lead ECG (*Fig. 1.29*).

ST segment depression that is maximal in leads V5 and V6 may also be related either to limited and transient ischaemia in the apex and septum of the left ventricle or to acute ischaemia of the right ventricle. It is the reciprocal effect to the elevation in leads V1 and V3 and V3R in lateral, transmural regional ischaemia (*Fig. 1.30*). Conversely, ST segment depression in leads V1 through V3 is often reflected by ST-segment elevation in leads V5 and V6.

Certain patients may manifest different forms of ischaemia at different times, varying from regional to circumferential ischaemia and from subendocardial to transmural ischaemia (*Figs 1.31, 1.32*). To recognize the different types of ischaemia, all the events that are accompanied by pain should be recorded during the period of hospitalization in the coronary care unit. The ECG may serve to reveal the culprit artery (*Fig. 1.33*).

PHASE II OF ACUTE ISCHAEMIA

Acute ischaemia differs from myocardial infarction in that in the former there is restoration of balance between oxygen supply and demand. The second phase of the ischaemic process is therefore the restoration of the supply–demand balance.

The changes occurring during this phase are determined by the type of changes that occurred during the first phase of the ischaemic process (*Fig. 1.34*). This phase may last from 20 minutes to 2 hours

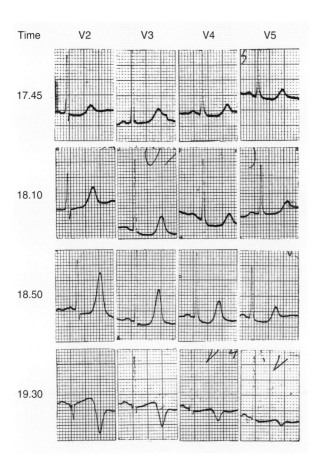

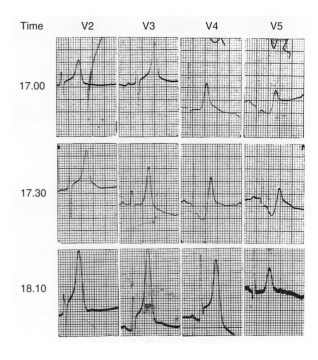

Figure 1.28 *Acute subendocardial regional ischaemia (17.00 and 17.30) evolving by 18.10 to transmural regional ischaemia.*

Figure 1.27 *Typical pattern of subendocardial regional ischaemia at 18.50, culminating in a characteristic ECG pattern of infarction (discussed in subsequent chapters) at 19.30.*

depending on the initial pathophysiology. In cases of transmural ischaemia, this process culminates in the inversion of the T wave in the affected leads (*Fig. 1.35*). If the T wave does not invert, the restoration process is not completed (*Fig. 1.36*), and thus the patient may be considered at higher risk (*Fig. 1.37*). In subendocardial ischaemia, the process may culminate in either inverted or upright T waves (*Figs 1.38, 1.39*). In contrast to transmural ischaemia, in subendocardial ischaemia the persistent presence of upright T waves does not indicate a worse prognosis (*Fig. 1.40*).

PHASE III OF ACUTE ISCHAEMIA

This phase encompasses the ECG changes occurring several days after the acute ischaemic event. These changes relate only to regional myocardial ischaemia. The author has noted a normalization process entailing four different scenarios in the configuration of the T waves (*Fig. 1.41*):

(a) Progressive normalization of the T wave from inverted to upright (*Fig. 1.42*). This usually takes 4–5 days.
(b) Pseudonormalization during a recurring ischaemic event, manifested by an acutely upright T wave that was previously inverted (*Fig. 1.43*).
(c) Persistently upright T waves (*Fig. 1.44*). These usually represent arteries that had not undergone complete reperfusion.
(d) Persistently negative T waves lasting more than 7 days (*Fig. 1.45*). These reflect residual subendocardial injury.

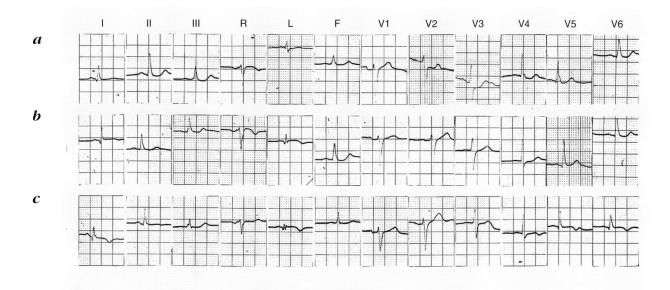

Figure 1.29 *(a) ST segment depression in leads V2 and V3 recorded during precordial pain. (b) Disappearance of pain; the ST segment becomes isoelectric in leads V2 and V3. Posterolateral wall infarction after 72 hours.*

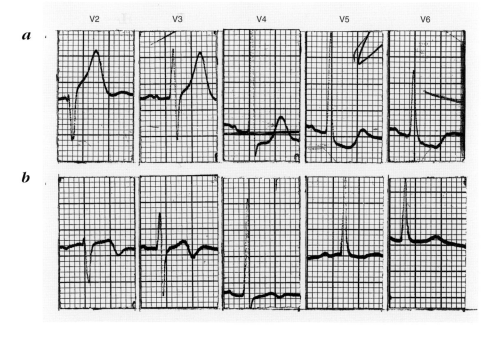

Figure 1.30 *Reciprocal ECG changes. (a) The tracing was obtained during pain, reflecting anteroseptal ischaemia. The ST-segment depression in leads V5 and V6 are reciprocal changes. The patient had ST segment elevation in leads V2 and V3 and ST segment depression in leads V5 and V6. (b) Two days later the T wave became inverted in leads V2 and V3, together with the resolution of the ST segment elevation. The ST segment depression resolved also. The inversion of the T wave in leads V2 and V3 reflect the natural course of ischaemia resolution, accompanied by the disappearance of reciprocal changes.*

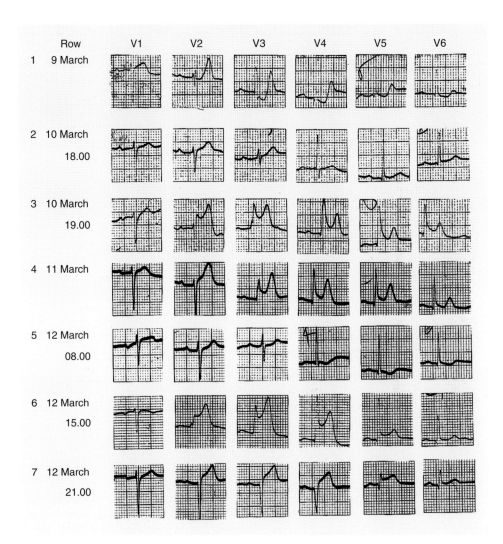

Figure 1.31 *Episodes of acute regional subendocardial ischaemia (top row), followed by acute transmural ischaemia (rows 3 and 4). In row 5, acute circumferential subendocardial ischaemia is evident. Row 6 depicts another episode of ischaemia. Eventually, the patient developed extensive anterior wall infarction with ST segment elevation (row 7).*

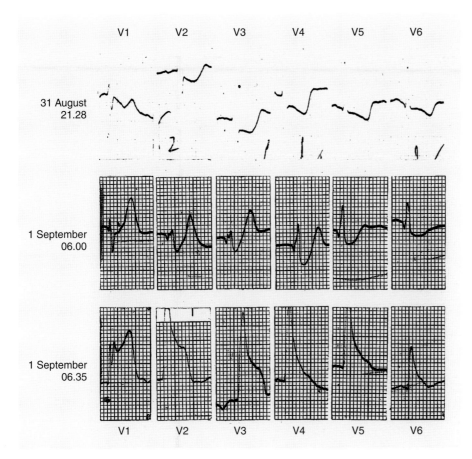

Figure 1.32   *The top row depicts acute circumferential subendocardial ischaemia. The middle row demonstrates Grade 3 acute regional subendocardial ischaemia in the same patient. The last row shows Grade 3 acute transmural ischaemia just before the patient's death.*

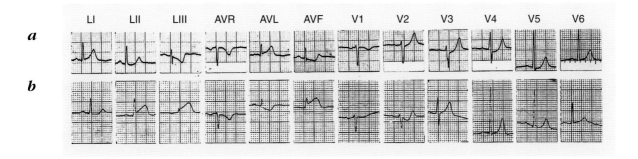

Figure 1.33   *An example of different culprit arteries in the same patient. (a) The ECG manifestations of acute ischaemia related to the circumflex artery. (b) ECG changes due to ischaemia in the regions subtended by the right coronary artery, occurring some 5 months later.*

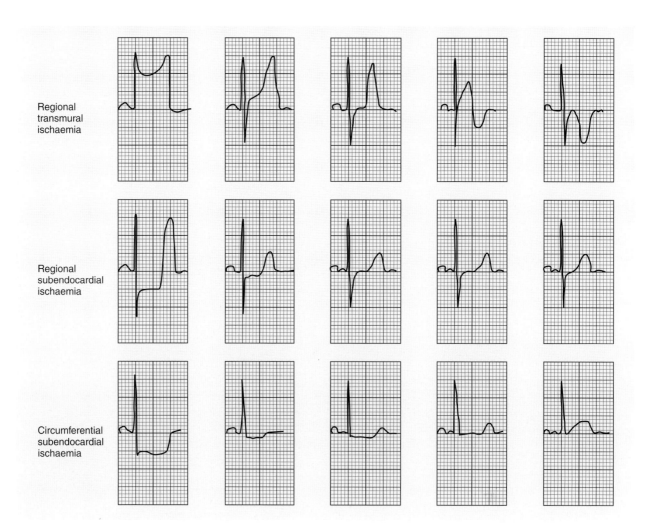

Figure 1.34   *Phase 2 of the different types of ischaemia.*

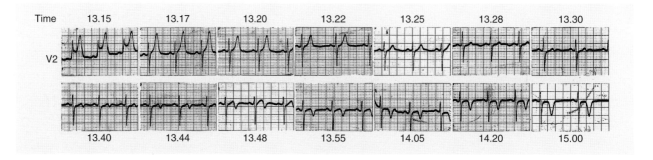

Figure 1.35   *Gradual ECG changes denoting the restoration of the balance in the ischaemic myocardium during Phase 2, culminating in the resolution of ST segment elevation and inverted T waves.*

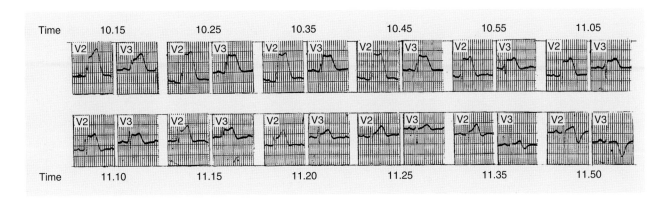

Figure 1.36 *Phase 2 of ischaemia after Grade 3 acute regional transmural ischaemia in Phase 1. Note that whereas the T wave is inverted in the last complex of lead V2 with slight ST segment elevation, there is no ST segment elevation in lead V3.*

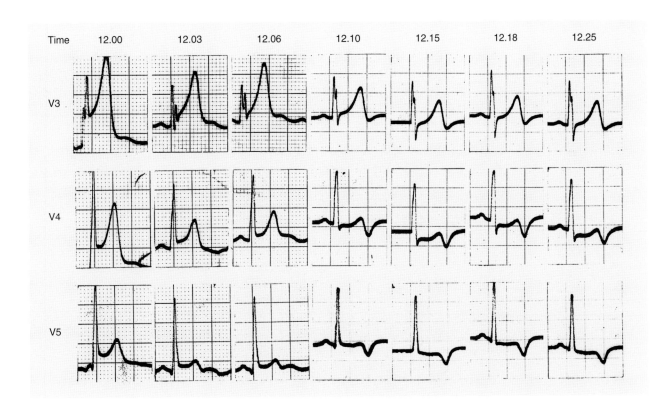

Figure 1.37 *The three-channel tracings were obtained simultaneously from the same patient during one episode of ischaemia. The different patterns of resolution of ECG changes in the different precordial leads, ranging from complete resolution of ST segment elevation to persistent ST segment elevation, and from upright to inverted T waves.*

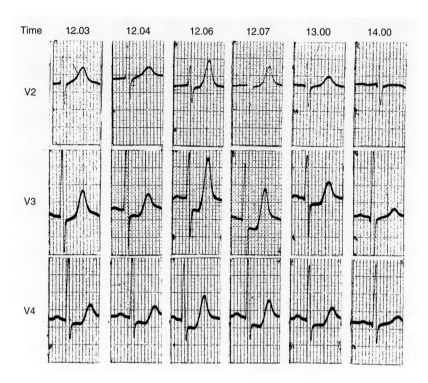

Figure 1.38 *Resolution of regional subendocardial ischaemia. The T waves in the last complex are upright.*

In the personal experience of the author, identifying these patterns is of therapeutic and prognostic significance. Pattern (a) (listed above) probably reflects the restoration of cell metabolism, a process that has been termed 'cellular recharging'. Thus, the ECG follows the metabolic changes.

Pattern (b) represents re-ischaemia; although the T wave becomes upright, the acute onset represents pseudonormalization, and not the normal process as in pattern (b). This pattern may or may not be accompanied by angina.

Pattern (c) represents incomplete reperfusion (thrombolysis in myocardial infarction (TIMI) flow 1–2). If TIMI flow is restored during subsequent coronary angioplasty, the T wave will invert after 20–30 minutes.

Pattern (d) probably represents incomplete 'recharging', due to more extensive damage to the myocardium.

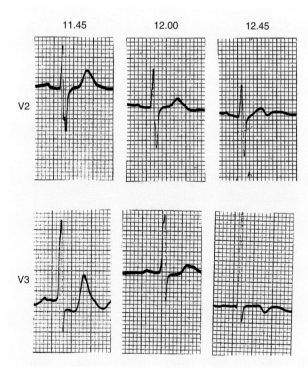

Figure 1.39 *Regional subendocardial ischaemia culminating in an inverted T wave in leads V2 and V3.*

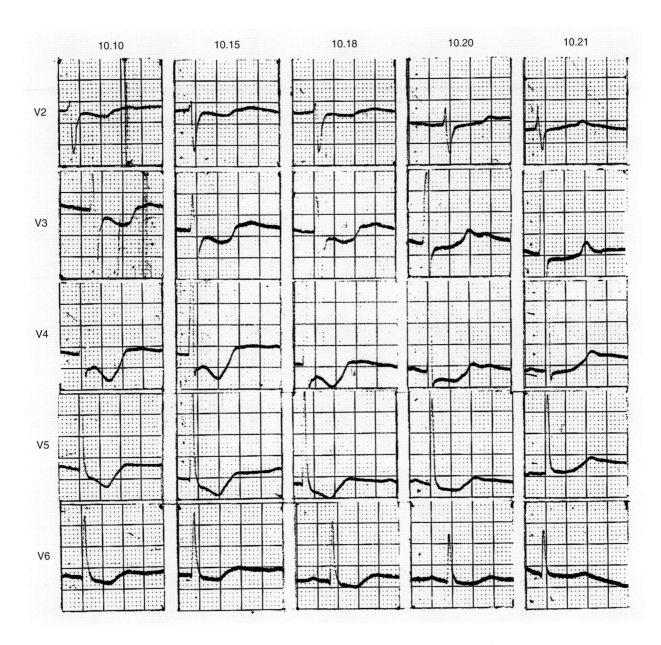

Figure 1.40 *Resolution of circumferential subendocardial ischaemia, culminating in upright T waves.*

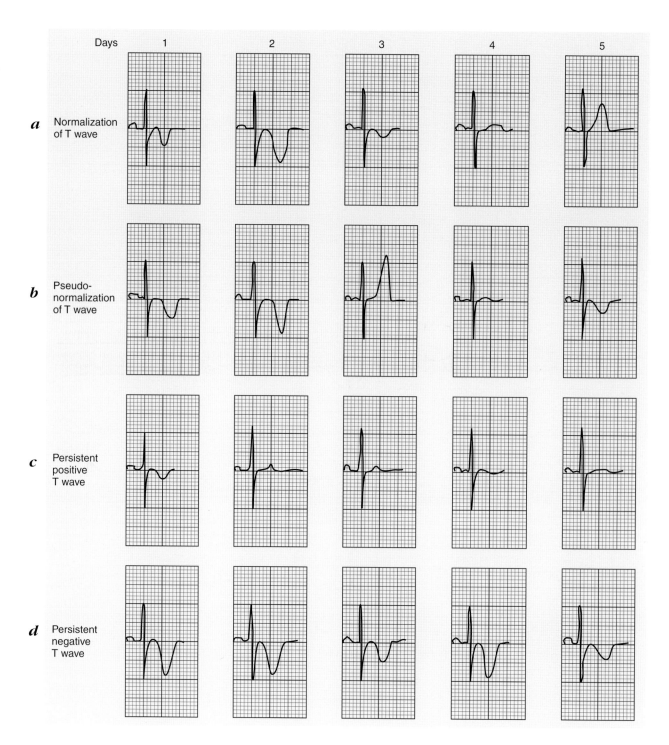

Figure 1.41 *The four different ECG types of Phase 3.*

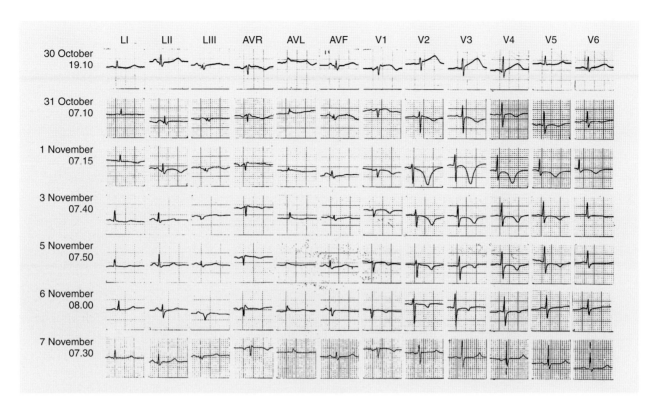

Figure 1.42 *ECG showing progressive normalization of the T wave over 7 days after ischaemia.*

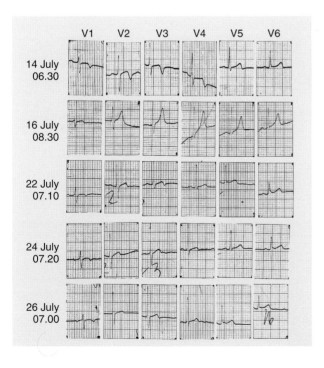

Figure 1.43 *ECG demonstrating that during the recovery after acute ischaemia there is acute pseudonormalization of the T wave (second row) during recurrent ischaemia.*

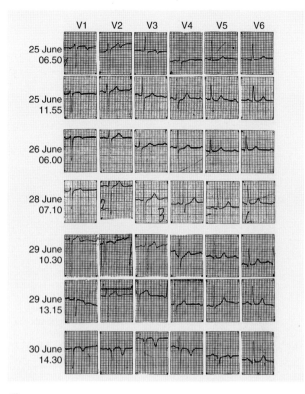

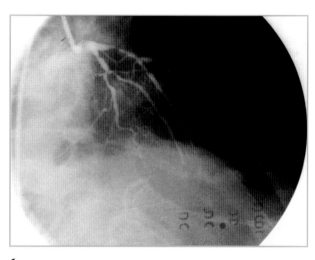

a   *b*

Figure 1.44 *(a) ECG tracings obtained during different days and hours in the same patient, showing different amplitudes of the T wave. Eventually, in the bottom row, anterior wall infarction was evident by ECG. (b) There is severe stenosis of the left anterior descending coronary artery with poor flow. The poor flow is reflected by the lack of T wave inversions in the involved leads.*

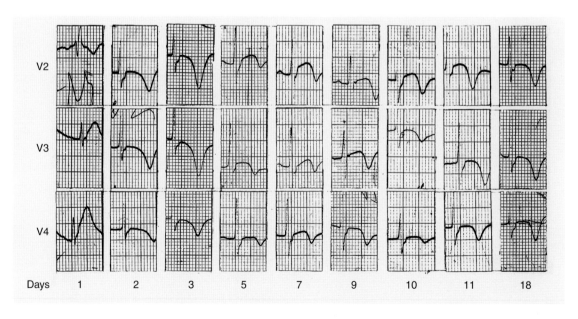

Figure 1.45 *ECG showing persistent inverted T waves over 18 days.*

REFERENCES

1. Braunwald E. Unstable angina. *Circulation* 1989; **80:**410–414.
2. Braunwald E, Jones RH, Mark DB et al, Diagnosis and managing of unstable angina. *Circulation* 1994; **90:**613–22.
3. Cohn PF. Total ischemic burden: pathophysiology and prognosis. *Am J Cardiol* 1987; **59:**30–6.
4. Chesebro JH, Zolhelyi P, Fuster V. Pathogenesis of thrombosis in unstable angina. *Am J Cardiol* 1991; **68:**B2–B10.
5. Lucas A, Antzelevich CH. Differences in the electrophysiological response of canine ventricular epicardium and endocardium in ischemia. *Circulation* 1993; **88:**2903–75.
6. Masseri A, Mimo R, Cherchia S, et al. Coronary artery spasm: a cause of acute myocardial ischemia in man. *Chest* 1975; **68:**625–33.
7. Ganz W. Coronary spasm in myocardial infarction fact or fiction? *Circulation* 1984; **63:**487–8.
8. Murrey CE, Jennigs RB, Reimer KA. Preconditioning with ischaemia: a delay in lethal cell injury in ischemic myocardium. *Circulation* 1986; **74:**1124–36.
9. Habib GD, Heibig J, Forman SA, et al. Influence of coronary collateral vessels on myocardial infarct size in human. *Circulation* 1991; **83:**739–46.
10. Sclarovsky S, Davidson E, Strasberg B, et al. Unstable angina: the significance of ST segment elevation or depression in patients without evidence of increased myocardial oxygen demand. *Am Heart J* 1986; **112:**463–7.
11. Sclarovsky S, Bassevich R, Strasberg B, et al. Unstable angina with tachycardia: clinical and therapeutical implications. *Am Heart J* 1988; **118:**1188–92.
12. Grossman W. Why is the left ventricle diastolic pressure increased during angina pectoris? *Am J Coll Cardiol* 1985; **5:**607–8.
13. Sclarovsky S, Davidson E, Strasberg B, et al. Unstable angina pectoris evolving to acute myocardial infarction: significance of ECG changes during chest pain. *Am Heart J* 1986; **112:**462.
14. Sambuceti G, Marzullo P, Giorgette A, et al. Global alteration in perfusion response to increasing oxygen consumption in patients with single vessel coronary artery disease. *Circulation* 1994; **90:**1696–1705.
15. Indolfi C, Ross J. The role of heart rate in myocardial ischemia and infarction: implication of myocardial perfusion–contraction matching. *Prog Cardiovasc Dis* 1993; **36:**64–74.
16. Indolfi C, Guth BD, Myazaki S, et al. Heart rate reduction improves myocardial ischemia in swine: role of interventricular blood flow redistribution. *Am J Physiol* 1991; **261:**H910–H917.
17. Sclarovsky S, Rechavia E, Strasberg B, et al. Unstable angina: ST segment with positive vs negative T wave. *Am Heart J* 1988; **116:**933–41.
18. Guyton R, McClenathan JH, Newman G, et al. Significance of subendocardial ST segment elevation caused by coronary stenosis in dog. Epicardial ST depression, local ischemia and subsequent necrosis. *Am J Cardiol* 1977; **40:**373–80.
19. Orchard CH, Kentish JC. Effects of changes in pH on the contractile function of cardiac muscle. *Am J Physiol* 1990; **258:**967–81.
20. Holland R, Brook H. The QRS complex during myocardial ischemia. *J Clin Invest* 1976; **57:**541–50.
21. Sclarovsky S, Topaz O, Rechavia E, et al. Ischemic ST segment depression in leads V2–V3 as the presenting ECG feature of posterolateral wall myocardial infarction. *Am Heart J* 1987; **113:**1085–90.

Chapter 2   Acute ischaemic syndrome—the pre-infarction ischaemic syndrome

SUMMARY

Pre-infarct syndrome is the initial ECG manifestation of acute ischaemia. It occurs before the development of acute infarction. It is important to identify the distinct ECG characteristics at this window of opportunity before irreversible myocardial damage develops. This chapter describes unique ECG patterns that are suggestive of:

- the site of occlusion;
- the coronary anatomy of the culprit artery as well as other coronary arteries; and
- the underlying myocardial milieu.

INTRODUCTION

The acute coronary syndrome comprises four clinical scenarios:[1]

- unstable angina;
- non-Q wave infarction;
- Q wave infarction;
- sudden death.

These four clinical scenarios have a common pathophysiological mechanism: transient or permanent obstruction, either mechanical or functional, of an epicardial artery.[2] The ECG can detect the transition of an ischaemic syndrome from transient ischaemia to an established infarct. This intermediate clinical picture has the same ECG characteristics as the acute ischaemias described in Chapter 1; however, in contrast to the transient obstruction in these acute ischaemias, the sudden coronary obstruction persists in the intermediate scenario. In the absence of reperfusion therapy (either pharmacological or mechanical), the ischaemic syndrome will culminate in acute infarction. Therefore the name 'pre-infarction syndrome' is appropriate. In the past, the term pre-infarction was used for unstable angina, but it was abandoned when it was discovered that the majority of cases of unstable angina do not evolve towards infarction (*Fig. 2.1*).[3]

Pre-infarction syndrome evolves in over 80% of cases toward acute infarction. Lately, a group of investigators have named it 'the initial pattern of

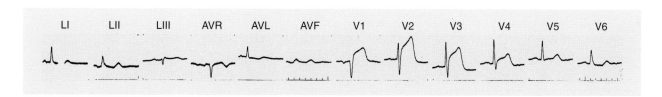

Figure 2.1   *Anterior wall pre-infarction syndrome. The precordial ST segment elevation is maximal in leads V2 and V3. The culprit artery is the left anterior descending artery, as was subsequently proved during coronary angiography. The culprit lesion was distal to the first diagonal branch. This was predicted before angiography, based on the absence of ST segment elevation in lead AVL. The mild ST segment elevation in lead LIII suggests that the LAD extends beyond the apex and subtends the inferior wall (a 'wrap-around' LAD). The ST segment elevation in lead V1 suggests that the left anterior descending artery also supplies the right aspect of the intraventricular septum. The ST segment depression in lead V6 represents a reciprocal change to the ST segment elevation in lead V1.*

acute myocardial infarction'.[4] However, the author of this book has elected to name this evolutionary stage of the acute ischaemic process 'pre-infarction syndrome', since most patients with this condition will evolve toward ECG or biochemical infarction. In similarity to the types of acute, transient ischaemia described in Chapter 1, three ECG subtypes of pre-infarction syndrome have been characterized:

- regional transmural pre-infarction ischaemia;
- regional subendocardial pre-infarction ischaemia;
- circumferential subendocardial pre-infarction ischaemia.

In this chapter, the ECG characteristics of the regional transmural pre-infarction syndrome will be discussed in detail. (The other two are discussed in Chapter 4.)

REGIONAL TRANSMURAL PRE-INFARCTION ISCHAEMIA

The syndrome is characterized by:

- pain lasting more than 30 minutes and up to 3–4 hours;
- positive and tall T waves;
- ST segment elevation;
- non Q waves or pathological Q waves that are not new.

From the therapeutic point of view, this clinical picture can be called 'the window of opportunity' before final regional infarction develops. Although patients with this picture have prolonged angina and ECG changes, they may not develop acute infarction, underscoring the need to intervene at this stage.

The ECG pattern of the regional transmural pre-infarction syndrome is determined by both anatomical factors (coronary and myocardial) and physiological factors (grade of ischaemia, which depends on the level of myocardial protection in the ischaemic area).

THE ECG AND ANATOMY DURING ANTERIOR WALL PRE-INFARCTION SYNDROME

From the ECG point of view the anterior wall of the left ventricle can be divided into two areas: the low anterior wall and the high anterior wall.

The low anterior wall projects its electric potentials toward the anteroposterior plane. It is shown in the ECG in the precordial leads V1 to V6 and it manifests the reciprocal potentials of the posterior and lateral wall. The high anterior area is manifested in the ECG in the frontal bipolar leads and in the unipolar leads of Wilson. The leads LI and AVL record the ischaemic potentials, and leads LIII and AVF represent the reciprocal potentials (*Fig. 2.2*).

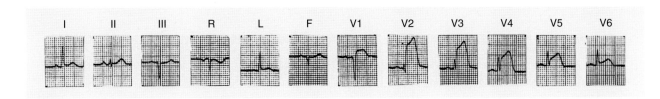

Figure 2.2 *Anterior wall pre-infarction syndrome. The precordial ECG changes encompass leads V2–V6, which suggests that the LAD subtends a substantial proportion of the anteroseptal and anterolateral walls. Although there is ST segment elevation in lead V1 there is no reciprocal change in lead V6 because of the ischaemia in the lateral wall. Moreover, the amplitude of the ST segment elevation is lower in leads V1 and V6, perhaps because of the attenuating effect of ischaemia in opposing walls. Note that despite the widespread precordial changes on the ECG, the frontal leads are not affected because the lesion in the left anterior descending artery is located distally, beyond the first diagonal.*

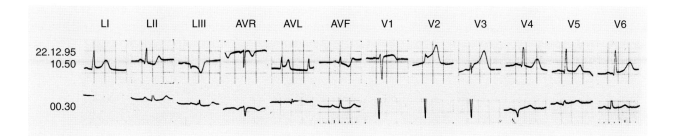

Figure 2.3 *Anterior wall pre-infarction syndrome. Note that the pattern of ST segment elevation is heterogenous in the different precordial leads, which suggests that the intensity of ischaemia varies in the different regions of the area at risk. In this case, the Grade 3 ischaemia in lead V2 suggests that it reflects the core of the ischaemia. Leads V3–V6 demonstrate the gradient in the intensity of ischaemia, as reflected by the gradual transition from Grade 2 ischaemia to Grade 1 (leads V4–V6). The fact that ischaemia Grade 3 is confined to one lead suggests that the core of ischaemia is not extensive. The ST segment elevation in lead AVL suggests that the lesion is in the proximal left anterior descending artery and that the ST segment depressions in leads LII, LIII, and AVF are reciprocal changes to the ST segment elevation in leads LI and AVL.*

Blood supply

The low anterior wall is nourished almost exclusively by the left anterior descending artery in the left paraseptal and apical region, and it is always represented in V2 and V3. (*Figs 2.1, 2.2, 2.3, 2.4*).

The lateral low anterior wall is supplied by a double circulation: the inferior diagonal branches of the left anterior descending artery and the marginal branches of the circumflex artery (*Fig. 2.5a*). This is why the lateral wall is spared in the majority of anterior infarcts (see *Figs 2.1, 2.2, 2.3*), and in most ischaemias of the lateral wall, the grade of ischaemia

is low (Grade 1). In the presence of a small circumflex artery or if the circumflex artery is occluded, the acute obstructions of the left anterior descending artery will present with more advanced signs of ischaemia in the low anterolateral leads (see *Figs 2.2, 2.5b*). If the circumflex artery and not the left anterior descending artery predominates, the circumflex artery will cause signs of severe ischaemia in the ECG from lead V6 toward V4 and even V3 (*Figs 2.5c, 2.6*).

The left inferior septal area is always supplied by the distal portion of the left anterior descending artery. Obstruction of this artery always causes

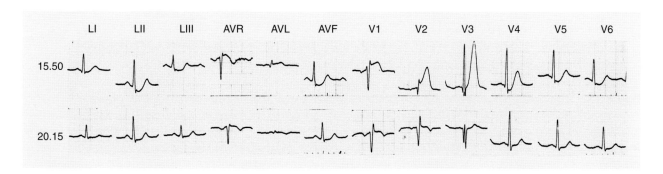

Figure 2.4 *Anterior wall pre-infarction syndrome. The maximal precordial changes in the ECG are localized to leads V2 and V3. However, the changes predominantly entail a change in the amplitude of the T wave rather than ST segment elevation. This type of ischaemia in lead V3 is classified as Grade 1. ST-segment elevation in lead V1 indicates involvement of the right ventricle. ST-segment depression in lead V6 is a reciprocal change. The bottom row depicts the ECG pattern after the resolution of the acute phase.*

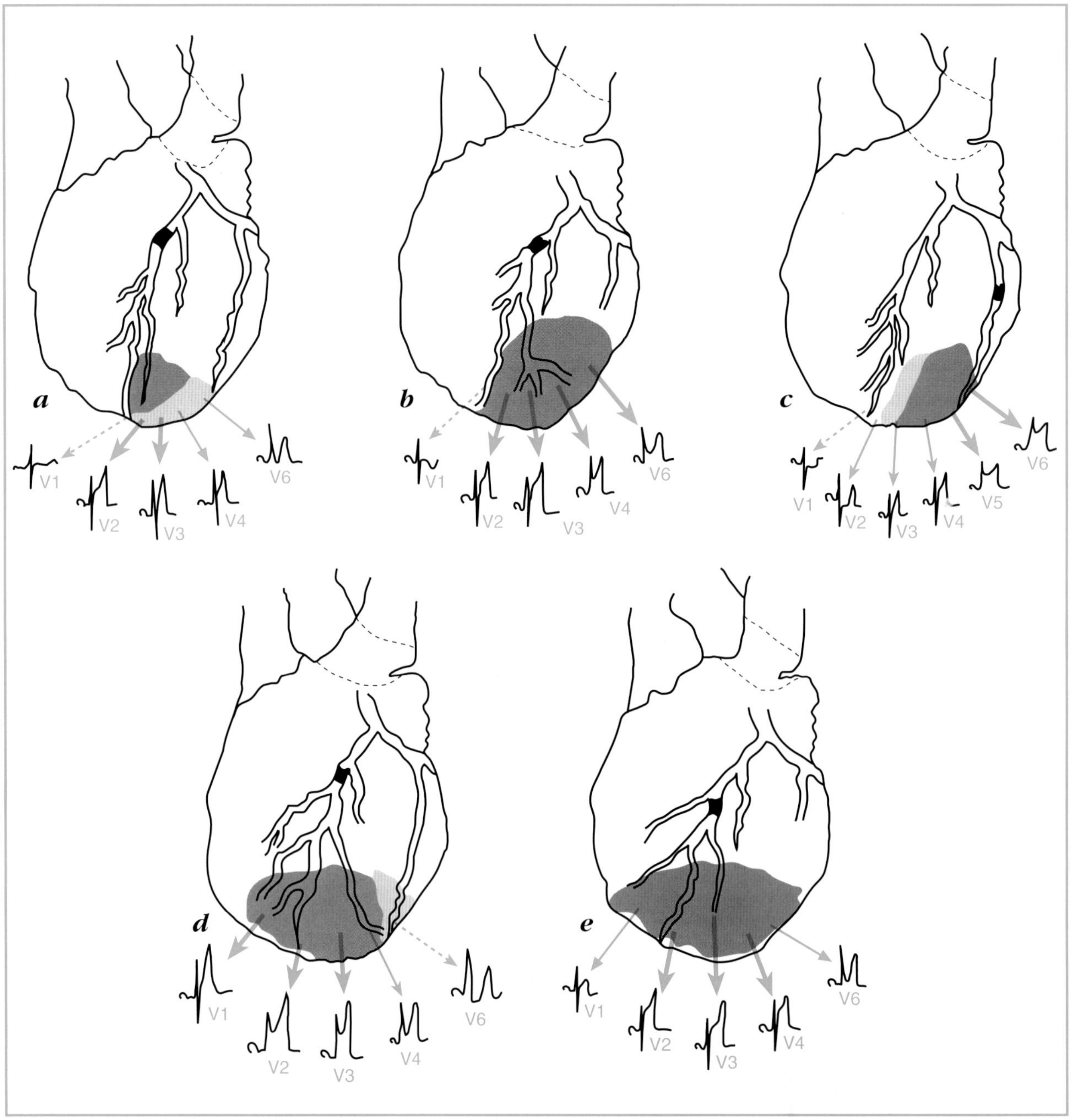

Figure 2.5 *A schematic illustration of the correlation between coronary anatomy and the ECG (anteroposterior projection). (a) An occluded LAD. The dots depict the border zone, whereas the diagonal lines depict the core of ischaemia. The border zone is shown in leads V5 and V6 with positive T waves. The core is subtended by leads V2–V4, and has the most dramatic changes in the ECG. (b) The LAD supplies the apical and lateral walls but not the right side of the septum. There is no attenuation, and thus the changes span all the way to V6. (c) An occluded circumflex marginal branch. The core of ischaemia is manifested in leads V5 and V6, whereas V1 manifests reciprocal changes. Leads V2 and V3 show lesser degrees of ischaemia, being the border zones. (d) The LAD supplies the right side of the septum and the lateral wall is supplied by the marginal branch. Lead V1 is not attenuated by leads V5 and V6, producing significant changes in V1. Lead V6 shows reciprocal changes to those evident in V1. (e) An occluded LAD without a marginal branch supplying the lateral wall. Note that the left anterior descending coronary artery supplies the right side of the septum. There are two opposite areas of ischaemia, and thus the changes in V1 and V6 are attenuated. The maximal grade of ischaemia is evident in leads V2–V5.*

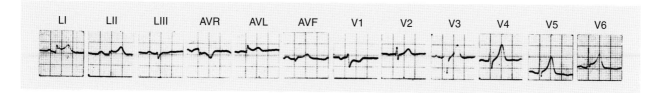

Figure 2.6 *An example of precordial ST segment elevation not caused by ischaemia related to the LAD. There is ST segment elevation in leads V3–V6, which is maximal in lead V6 and minimal in lead V3. Note the absence of ST segment elevation in lead V2. The limb leads demonstrate ST segment elevation in leads LI and AVL, suggesting involvement of the first marginal branch of the left circumflex coronary artery. Note also the ST segment elevation in lead LII, and the absence of such changes in lead LIII, suggesting that LII reflects the ischaemia in the posterolateral wall.*

maximum ischaemia in the left paraseptal and apical zone and in leads V2 and V3 (see *Figs 2.1, 2.2, 2.3, 2.4, 2.5a–d*).

The right area of the septum has a double circulation, the left anterior descending artery and the conal branch of the right coronary artery. Lead V1 shows the ECG changes caused by ischaemia in the right side of the septum (*Figs 2.5d,e, 2.7*). However, when the circulation of the right septum is supplied predominantly by the left anterior descending artery and an acute obstruction of this artery occurs, the ECG will show pronounced elevation of the ST segment in lead V1 (*Fig. 2.8a*). When most of the right septum is supplied by the right conal artery, the T

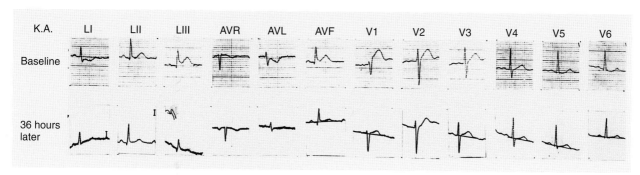

a

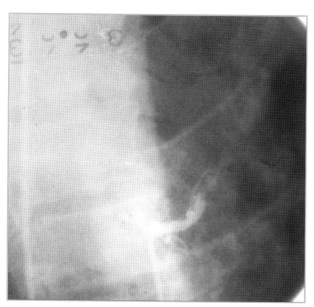

b

Figure 2.7 *(a) An ECG showing an example of precordial ST segment elevation not caused by ischaemia related to the LAD. The precordial ST segment elevation in this case represents right ventricular infarction. This is suggested by the maximal precordial ST segment elevation in lead V1, and the concomitant changes in the inferior leads. (b) An angiogram showing the culprit artery was the right coronary artery in its proximal portion. This type of ischaemia should be distinguished from the anteroinferior ischaemias caused by a large LAD extending beyond the apex and subtending the inferior wall. In that case, the maximal ST segment elevation would be in leads V2 and V3 (see Fig. 2.16).*

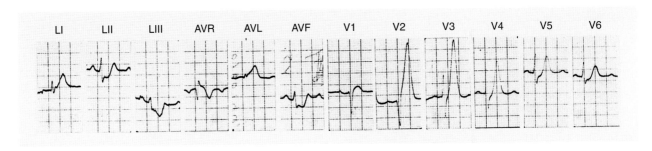

Figure 2.8 *An example of anterior wall pre-infarct syndrome accompanied by right ventricular septal involvement. This is reflected by ST segment elevation in leads V1 and V3R (a). This is in contrast to anterior wall pre-infarct syndrome without right ventricular septal involvement (b). In this case, there is no ST segment elevation in lead V1 and VR3. Note that in both cases the precordial ST segment elevation is in leads V2 and V3, reflecting involvement of the LAD.*

Figure 2.9 *Anterior wall pre-infarct syndrome caused by involvement of the first diagonal branch. ST segment elevation with upright T waves in leads AVL, LI, and V2 are noted. The involvement of these three leads together suggests that the diagonal branch is the culprit artery. Leads V3–V6 manifest tall, peaked T waves with ST segment depression, suggesting subendocardial regional ischaemia of the anterolateral wall. Reciprocal changes are noted in inferior leads (LIII and AVF); these entail ST segment depression with inverted T waves.*

waves in lead V1 remain inverted and the ST segment remains isoelectric (see *Fig. 2.8b*).[5]

The high anterior wall is supplied by three arteries: the first diagonal artery (D1), the intermediate artery, and the first marginal of the circumflex artery (M1). Acute and persistent obstruction of one of these arteries will cause ST segment elevation and upright T waves in AVL, and ST segment depression and inverted T waves (reciprocal effects) in lead LIII (*Fig. 2.9*).[6]

ANALYSIS OF THE ECG

Systematic analysis of the ECG pattern in the pre-infarction ischaemic syndrome can provide anatomical, pathophysiological, and prognostic data.

ANATOMICAL ANALYSIS

Anatomical analysis can be carried out:

- at the level of the coronary arteries; and
- at the myocardial level.

When analysing the anatomy of the coronary arteries, the following parameters are considered:

- the culprit artery;
- the level of obstruction; and
- the dimensions of the culprit artery.

The culprit artery in anterior infarcts

The low anterior wall is supplied exclusively by the left anterior descending artery. Therefore, one may readily diagnose an obstruction of the left anterior descending artery in anterior infarcts, because the maximal changes in the ECG (the core of the ischaemia) are evident in leads V2 and V3. But sometimes the low anterior wall is nourished by another artery that is oriented forward; for example, the marginals of the circumflex or the marginals of the right coronary artery. Obstruction of these arteries is seen in the precordial leads, but it never causes maximal changes in leads V2 and V3 (see *Figs 2.5c, 2.6, 2.7*).

The level of obstruction

In contrast to earlier studies, which divided the left anterior descending artery based on the septal branches, the author has determined the level of obstruction of the left anterior descending artery by its relationship with the first diagonal artery.[7] If the obstruction is located above the first diagonal artery, it is considered proximal. If the obstruction is located below it, it is considered distal.

The first diagonal artery supplies the high anterior wall: when this wall is ischaemic because of an acute obstruction of this artery, there will commonly be ST segment elevation with positive T waves in AVL, and ST segment depression with inverted T waves in lead LIII (*Figs 2.9, 2.10*). ST segment elevation in AVL may be accompanied neither by ST segment elevation in lead LI nor by ST segment depression in leads AVF and LII.

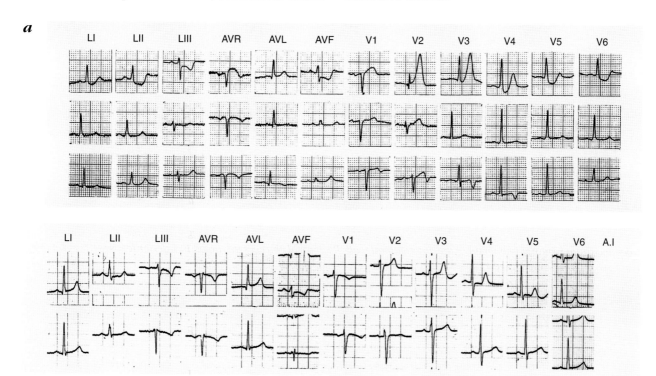

Figure 2.10   *Serial ECG tracings obtained every 24 hours showing diagonal artery obstruction. (a) Pre-infarction syndrome of the mid-anterior wall of the left ventricle. Note the ST segment elevation in leads AVL and V2 with positive T waves; ST segment depression in leads LIII and AVF with inverted T waves; ST segment depression in leads V3, V4, and V5 with peaked and tall T waves. (b) The same ECG pattern in another patient. In (a) the ischaemia developed with ECG signs of acute infarction whereas in (b) the ischaemia resolved without subsequent ECG changes of infarction.*

Acute obstruction of the left anterior descending artery

The ECG pattern of the frontal leads in anterior infarction is determined by two factors: the level of obstruction and whether or not the apex of the left ventricle is subtended by the left anterior descending artery ('wrap-around' left anterior descending artery).

Therefore, four conditions are recognized:

No wrapping of the left anterior descending artery
- Proximal: Lead AVL: ST segment elevation and positive T waves;
  Lead LIII: ST segment depression and negative T waves (*Figs 2.11b, 2.12*).

- Distal: Lead AVL: isoelectric ST segment;
  Lead LIII: isoelectric ST segment (*Figs 2.11a, 2.13*).

Wrapping of the left anterior descending artery
- Proximal: Lead AVL: moderately elevated, positive T waves;
  Lead LIII: moderately depressed, positive T waves (*Figs 2.11d, 2.14, 2.15*).

- Distal: Lead AVL: ST segment depression and inverted T waves;
  Lead LIII: ST segment elevation and positive T waves (*Figs 2.11c, 2.16*).

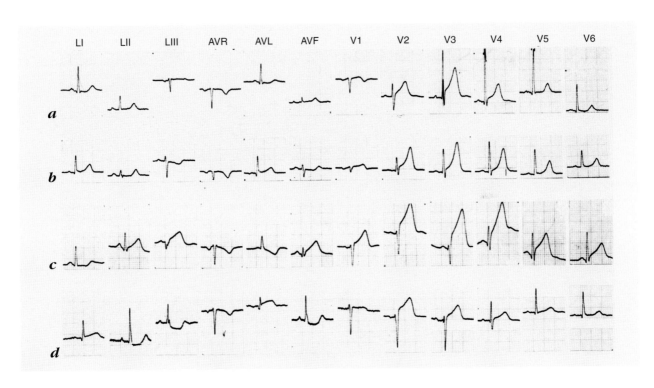

Figure 2.11 *The use of the limb leads to localize the culprit lesion (level of obstruction) in the left anterior descending artery. (a) Ischaemia Grade 2 is noted in precordial leads, but the limb leads are spared, suggesting that the obstruction is in the distal left anterior descending artery, and that the LAD (type B) again does not extend beyond the apex.*
(b) Ischaemia Grade 2 is noted in the precordial leads, and the concomitant ST segment elevation in lead AVL and the ST segment depression in leads LIII and AVF (with inverted T waves) suggest that the LAD (type B) lesion is in its proximal part, and that the artery does not extend beyond the apex. (c) Ischaemia Grade 2 is seen in the precordial leads. Note, ST-segment elevation and positive T-waves in lead L3 and in lead AVF as well; lead AVL shows ST-segment depression with negative T-waves. This pattern suggests a distal obstruction type C of the left anterior descending artery. (d) Ischaemia Grade 2 is noted in the precordial leads, with ST segment elevation in lead AVL, and ST segment depression in leads LIII and AVF. In contrast to (a), the ST segment depression in leads LIII and AVF is accompanied by upright T waves, suggesting the lesion is in the proximal left anterior descending artery, and that the LAD (type C) extends beyond the apex.

a

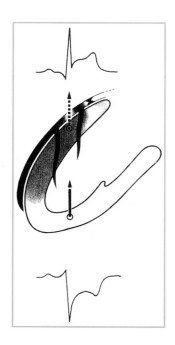

Figure 2.12   *A case of a proximal lesion in the LAD, which does not extend beyond the apex. (a) Diagram depicting the site of involvement in the LAD, the extent of the LAD relative to the apex, and the concomitant ECG changes. Note the ST segment elevation with upright T waves in the anterolateral leads, and the ST segment depression with inverted T waves in the inferior leads. The dotted arrow depicts the injury vector, whereas the bold arrow denotes the reciprocal vector. (b) Twelve-lead ECG from a patient with this lesion. (c) Coronary angiography before angioplasty confirmed the proximal location of the stenosis. The arrow points to the site of obstruction. (d) After angioplasty, the LAD was shown to extend up to the apex but not beyond.*

b

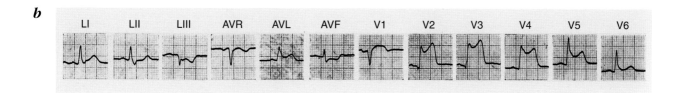

c

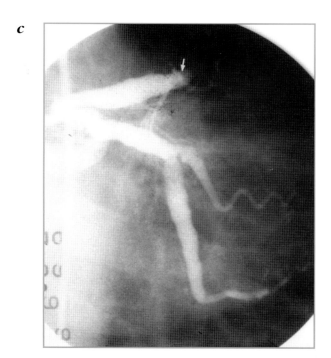

d

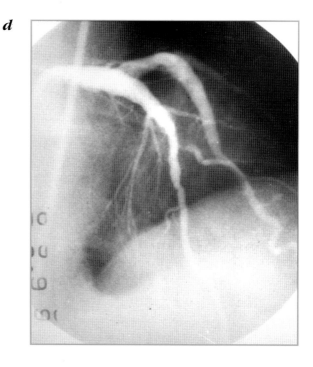

a

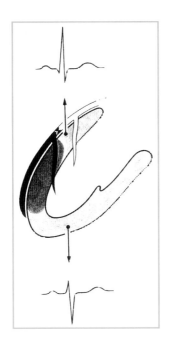

Figure 2.13 *A case of a distal lesion in the LAD, which does not extend beyond the apex. (a) Diagram depicting the site of involvement in the LAD, the extent of the LAD relative to the apex, and the concomitant ECG changes. Note the ST segment elevation with upright T waves in the anterior leads, and the lack of changes in the inferior and lateral leads. The two opposing arrows depict the vectors of depolarization without an injury pattern. (b) Twelve-lead ECG from a patient with this lesion. (c) Coronary angiography before angioplasty confirmed the distal location of the stenosis (distal to first diagonal). After angioplasty, the LAD was shown to extend up to the apex but not beyond (not shown).*

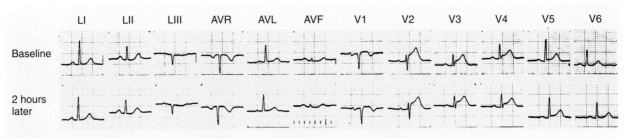

b

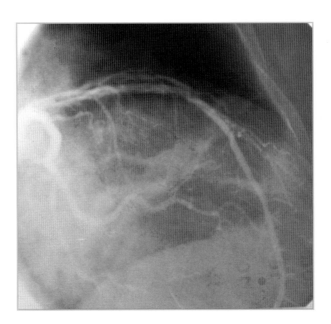

c

a

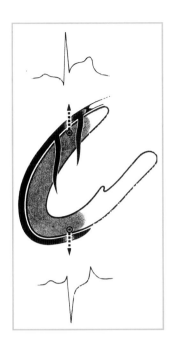

Figure 2.14   *A case of a proximal lesion in the LAD, which extends beyond the apex. (a) Diagram depicting the site of involvement in the LAD, the extent of the LAD relative to the apex, and the concomitant ECG changes. Note the ST segment elevation with upright T waves in the anterolateral leads, and the ST segment depression with upright T waves in the inferior leads. The dotted arrows depict the injury vector. Note that the arrows are small, denoting the attenuation of the injury vector by the two opposing vectors. (b) Twelve-lead ECG from a patient with this lesion. (c) Coronary angiography after angioplasty of the proximal LAD confirmed the extent of the LAD beyond the apex.*

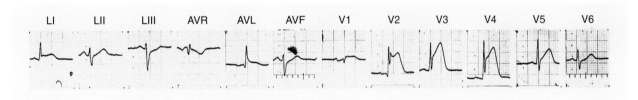

b

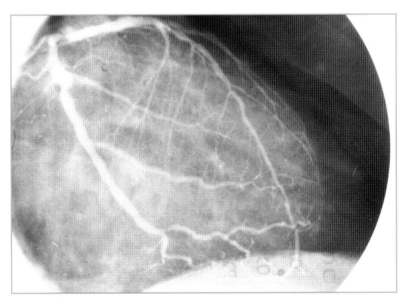

c

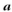

a

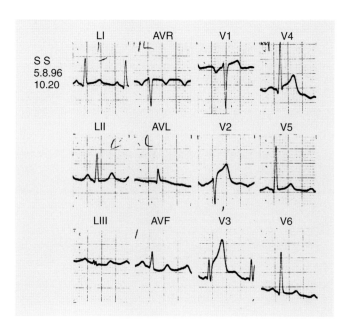

b

Figure 2.15 *Two more examples of proximal wrapping of the LAD. Note the moderate ST segment elevation in AVL (0.5 mm) with a flat T wave. In lead LIII there is mild ST segment depression (0.5 mm) with upright T waves. Note that in (b) the ST segment elevation and T waves are of greater amplitude in LI than they are in (a) in AVL.*

The dimensions of the culprit artery

The dimensions (length) can be determined by the number of ECG leads involved in the ischaemic process. By relating the dimensions of the left anterior descending artery (LAD) to the apex of the left ventricle, three sizes of this artery can be recognized:[8]

- Type A: the LAD does not reach the apex;
- Type B: the LAD reaches the apex;
- Type C: the LAD crosses beyond the apex.

When the artery is of type A, leads V2 and V3 are generally involved; lead V4 seldom is. Arteries of types B and C involve the whole low anterior wall, the left paraseptal and apical wall and the antero-lateral wall, and leads V2 and V6 are involved.

Leads V4 and V6 show signs of low-grade ischaemia (Grade 1 or 2). Ischaemia Grade 1 is not recognized as a sign of ischaemia (i.e. not readily appreciated by ECG unless the index of suspicion is high), but 30% of patients with it develop Q waves within 24–72 hours, and 80% develop inverted T waves. Ischaemia Grade 1 is probably due to the double circulation existing in the low anterolateral wall, as described above (*Figs 2.3, 2.5a*).

Arteries of type C also supply the inferior wall of the left ventricle. When the obstruction is distal in an artery of type C, ST segment elevation and upright T waves in leads LIII and AVF develop. The ECG of

a

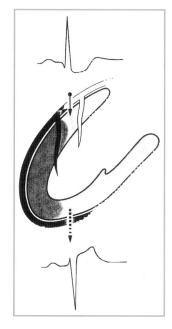

c

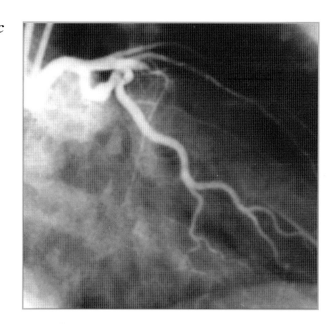

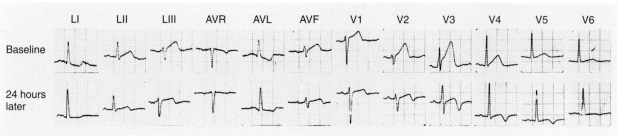

b

Figure 2.16 *A case of a distal lesion in the LAD, which extends beyond the apex. (a) Diagram depicting the site of involvement in the LAD, the extent of the LAD relative to the apex, and the concomitant ECG changes. Note the ST segment depression with inverted T waves in the anterolateral leads, and the ST segment elevation with upright T waves in the inferior leads. The dotted arrow depicts the injury vector, whereas the bold arrow denotes the reciprocal vector. (b) Twelve-lead ECG from a patient with this lesion. (c) Coronary angiography after angioplasty of the distal LAD confirmed the extent of the LAD beyond the apex.*

many patients with this phenomenon evolves towards Q waves in the posteroinferior leads (LIII and AVF) (see *Fig. 2.16*).[9]

The attenuation phenomenon

When the obstruction is proximal to the first diagonal artery of type C, the so-called 'attenuation phenomenon' occurs, in which the same artery supplies two electrically opposite areas (*Figs 2.15a,b*). Ischaemia develops in both the high anterior area and the inferoposterior area. Owing to the opposite orientation of these vectors, the signs of ischaemia and the reciprocal signs are attenuated. A slight depression of the ST segment and the slightly upright T waves are

observed in lead LIII, and the elevation of the ST segment in lead AVL is attenuated.

In the EGC of patients with an obstruction proximal to the diagonal artery and LAD of type B, the ST segment and the T waves in AVL will be higher than the ST segment and T waves in lead LI (see *Figs 2.3, 2.12*).

If the obstruction is proximal to the diagonal artery and LAD is of type C, the ST segment and the T waves in lead LI are higher than the ST segment and the T waves in AVL. This is the attenuation phenomenon (see *Figs 2.14, 2.15*).

The attenuation phenomenon is also seen in other arteries, such as the right coronary artery and the circumflex artery. An acute proximal occlusion of the

	LI	LII	LIII	AVR	AVL	AVF	V1	V2	V3	V4	V5	V6
Baseline												
24 hours later												

a

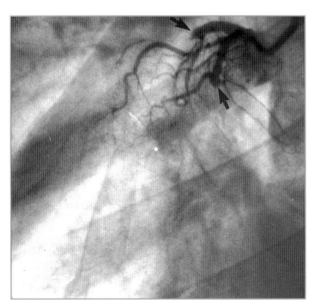

b

Figure 2.17 *(a) Acute anterior pre-infarct syndrome with an ECG tracing obtained 20 minutes after onset of symptoms (upper trace). Note the widespread ST segment elevation in precordial leads with Grade 3 ischaemia in leads V4–V6. This pattern suggests concomitant disease of the left circumflex coronary artery, although the culprit artery is the LAD. Lower trace describes the effective reperfusion signs immediately after angioplasty. (b) This was confirmed by coronary angiography. Both the LAD and the circumflex artery were obstructed distally. The culprit artery was identified by ECG; maximal precordial ST segment elevation in leads V2 and V3 suggests that the LAD is the culprit. After angioplasty of the LAD distal to the first diagonal branch, there were ECG signs of reperfusion.*

right coronary artery may induce ischaemia in two opposite areas, such as the right anteroseptal wall and the posterior wall. A proximal occlusion of the circumflex artery produces ischaemia in opposite areas, such as the high anterior and inferoposterior areas.

The left anterior descending artery sometimes supplies two different opposite areas, such as the right septum, represented in the ECG by lead V1, and the lateral wall, represented by leads V5 and V6 (see *Fig. 2.5e*). In most patients, ST segment elevation (over 2 mm) occurs in lead V1, together with ST segment depression in lead V6 (see *Figs 2.3, 2.5d*), indicating involvement of the lower lateral wall, unless ST segment depression in lead V6 is attenuated by an ischaemic process (see *Figs 2.2, 2.4*).

Myocardial anatomy

The ischaemia that occurs during the pre-infarct process in the myocardium is not uniform. There are zones that are more affected (the core of ischaemia), and the border zone, which is less affected. In obstructions of the left anterior descending artery, the core of the ischaemia will be seen in leads V2 and V3, V4 being a zone of transition between the core and the border zone (see *Figs 2.1, 2.2, 2.4*). The border zone is observed in leads V5 and V6 (*Fig. 2.18*). It can be recognized because of the low grade of ischaemia that results from the double circulation supplying this area (see *Fig. 2.18*). However, if the circumflex artery does not supply the anterolateral wall, the core of ischaemia will be very extensive (see *Figs 2.5b, 2.17*).

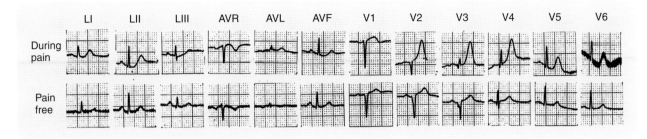

a

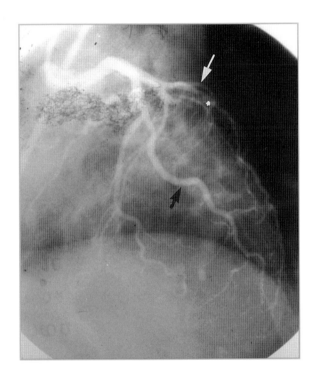

b

Figure 2.18   *(a) Pre-infarct syndrome of the anterior wall is manifested by maximal changes in leads V2 and V3. Note that there is no ST segment elevation from V3 to V6, although there are tall, peaked T waves (Grade 1 ischaemia). (b) Coronary angiogram from the patient whose ECG is shown in (a). Note the occluded left anterior descending coronary artery (white arrow) and the big marginal branch of the left circumflex coronary artery (black arrow) supplying the distal territory subtended by the left anterior descending coronary artery.*

PHYSIOLOGICAL FACTORS

The intensity of the ischaemia indicates the presence or absence of myocardial protection. The intensity is revealed by the grades of ischaemia, which are the same as described for the transient ischaemias (see Chapter 1).

Pre-infarct ischaemia Grade 3

This occurs in 30–40% of the patients with pre-infarct syndrome. Three morphologies of ischaemia Grade 3 can be recognized on the ECG by considering the relationship between the three systolic electrical components:

- the T waves;
- the ST segment;
- the degree of distortion of the terminal portion of the QRS complex and the increase in the size of R waves (see *Fig. 2.12*).

Pre-infarct syndrome with ischaemia Grade 3, type A
This type can be recognized by: positive and tall T waves; ST segment elevation with a terminal distortion of the QRS complex (ST segment generally does not cross the middle of the QRS complex); disappearance of the S waves and a slight increase in the

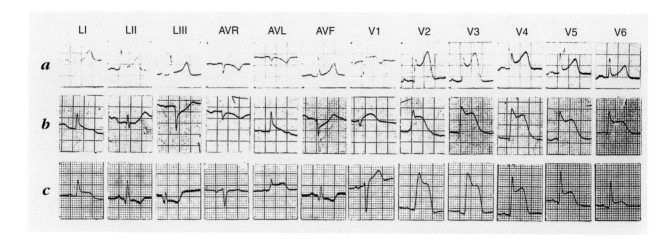

Figure 2.19 *The three different types of Grade 3 ischaemia. (a) The S wave disappears in leads V2 and V3, the ST segment is concave, and the T wave is greater in amplitude than the ST segment. (b) The S wave disappears, the ST segment is not concave, and the T wave is approximately of the same amplitude as the ST segment. (c) The S wave disappears, the ST segment is not concave, and the T wave is of lesser amplitude than the ST segment.*

R waves (*Fig. 2.19a*). The cause for this pattern appears to be the depression of the conducting system in the ischaemic area.[10]

Ischaemia Grade 3 type A may appear in one lead or two (see *Fig. 2.3*). When four or five leads are involved, it is presented as ischaemia Grade 3 type B or ischaemia Grade 3 type C, and it is considered severe.

Pre-infarct syndrome with ischaemia Grade 3, type B
This pattern is characterized in the ECG by ST segment elevation and upright T waves that are iso-electric with the ST segment, regardless of the amplitude of the R waves or the ST segment elevation (*Fig. 2.19b*). This pattern may be explained by the depression of phase 4 of the action potential.[11]

Pre-infarct syndrome with ischaemia Grade 3, type C
In this pattern, the ST segments are higher than the T waves and the QRS complex is increased in size (*Fig. 2.19c*). This pattern seems to be of more severe prognosis than the others.

A unique type of ischaemia Grade 3, type C has been noticed. A pattern of acute anterior pre-infarction characterized by ischaemia Grade 3 with maximal changes in leads V4 and V6 and a marked elevation of the ST segment with upright T waves in lead V2 but with a QS pattern is not uncommon. This pattern portends a poor clinical prognosis with high mortality rates and severe damage to the left ventricle. QS morphology in lead V2 indicates that the injury vector is displaced to the left (*Fig. 2.20*). This pattern has been explained by Silvester as a

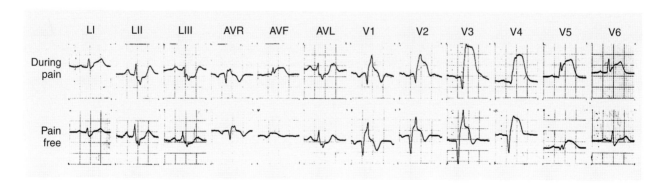

Figure 2.20 *Ischaemia Grade 3 in leads V4–V6 and ischaemia Grade 2 in leads V2 and V3. The lateral location of the ischaemia Grade 3 portends a very poor prognosis.*

sign of a severe depression of the septal Purkinje conductive system.[12]

Most patients with ischaemia Grade 3 type B or type C present with a tiny Q wave in leads V2 and V3. This Q wave may be due to an early necrosis of the subendocardial area.

It is known that animals that lack myocardial protection (e.g. pigs) develop Q waves very early when an epicardial artery is occluded,[13] whereas animals with myocardial protection (e.g. dogs) develop Q waves much later.[14] Most patients with ischaemia Grade 3 develop Q waves within 3 hours of the onset of pain.

Pre-infarct syndrome with ischaemia Grade 2

This pattern is characterized by:

- positive T waves;
- ST segment elevation of more than 2 mm;
- S waves below the reference segment PR or TR (*Fig. 2.21*).

Various subtypes of ischaemia Grade 2 can be recognized by taking into account the relationship between the T waves and the ST segment.

Pre-infarct syndrome with ischaemia Grade 2, type A
This type is characterized by

- tall T waves (approximately 15 mm);

- ST segments of approximately 2–3 mm;
- QRS complexes with no morphological changes (see *Fig. 2.21a*).

This type has the best clinical prognosis.

Pre-infarct syndrome with ischaemia Grade 2, type B
The ST segments and the T waves are of the same amplitude with no alteration in the S waves. The ST segments may become elevated up to 5–6 mm, and the T waves are of the same amplitude (see *Fig. 2.21b*). The author believes that ST segment elevation of 5 mm with T waves of 15 mm carries a different prognosis than the pattern of ischaemia Grade 2, type B with the ST segments and T waves of the same amplitude. This latter pattern may reveal a lack of epicardial protection, and most patients with anterior wall ischaemia and rupture of myocardium present with this pattern (*Fig. 2.22*).

Pre-infarct syndrome with ischaemia Grade 2, type C
This type is characterized by:

- ST segment elevation up to 12–13 mm;
- tall T waves (up to 15 mm);
- decrease in S waves (though they do not cross the reference line) (see *Fig. 2.21c*).

There is also an intermediate pattern between Grade 3 and Grade 2 in which the S waves are not totally erased and remain stagnant above the reference line.

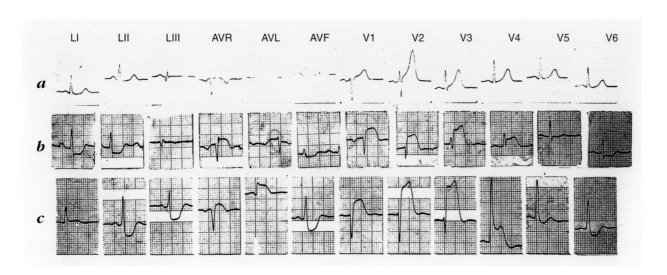

Figure 2.21 *Three examples of ischaemia Grade 2. (a) Tall, peaked T waves in leads V2 and V3 with moderate ST segment elevation. Note the difference between the amplitudes of the T wave and the ST segment. (b) The T wave is of the same amplitude as the ST segment. (c) Both the ST segment and the T waves are of great amplitude.*

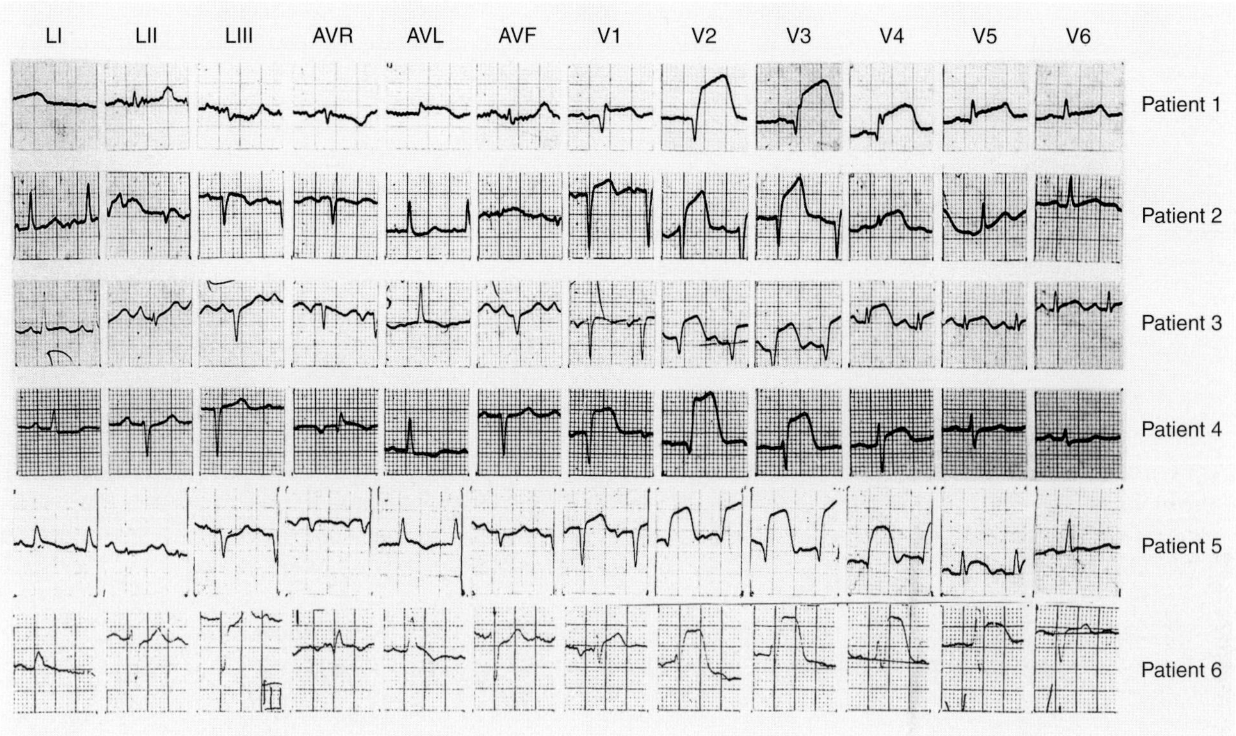

Figure 2.22 *ECG tracings during the pre-infarct syndrome from six consecutive patients who died from cardiac rupture (confirmed by echocardiography) after thrombolytic therapy. Note that all the patients had ischaemia Grade 2, with T wave of the same amplitude as the ST segment. Both T waves and the ST segments were of moderate height (type B).*

Pre-infarct syndrome with ischaemia Grade 1

This pattern is characterized by the development of peaked and tall T waves, with no elevation of the ST segment and with no distortion of the QRS complex.

Ischaemia Grade 1 must be considered in two clinical conditions. The first condition is that patients with acute pre-infarction syndrome develop ischaemia Grade 1 in the 'core' of the ischaemic process (leads V2 and V3).[15] The diagnosis of this type of infarct is overlooked in the Emergency Room because there is no ST segment elevation. Therefore, it is difficult to evaluate the incidence of these infarcts. This grade indicates the maximum level of myocardial protection conferred by the collateral circulation or other mechanisms (*Figs 2.18, 2.23*). These patients generally have a long history of stable angina caused by a severe chronic obstruction of an epicardial artery, and it is this that has allowed the evolution of a collateral circulation. Therefore, when the thrombus that completely occludes the artery develops, there already exists a 'prepared collateral circulation', giving the mycocardium maximal protection. These patients have been seen much less frequently in the past few years, probably because of angioplastic intervention in patients with stable or progressive angina.

The second clinical condition to be considered is the presence of ischaemia Grade 1 in the 'border zone' of an extensive pre-infarction syndrome. This is generally observed in leads V4–V6 owing to the protection effect of the double circulation of the anterolateral wall; however 30% of patients with ischaemia Grade 1 in leads V4 and V6 develop Q waves. In another 30%, a decrease in the magnitude of the R waves is recorded. In both conditions ischaemia Grade 1 is overlooked (see leads V5 and V6 in *Fig. 2.16*).

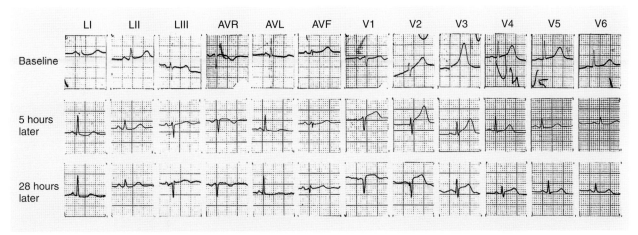

a

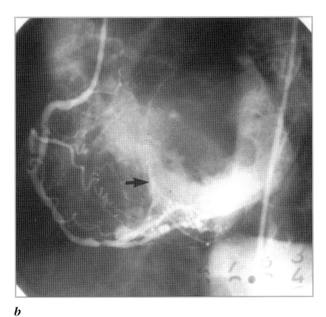

b

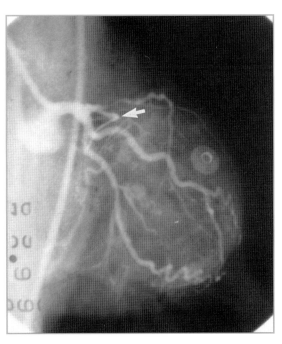

c

Figure 2.23   *(a) The ECG tracing shows maximal precordial changes in leads V2 and V3, ST segment elevation of 1 mm in leads V2 and V3 with tall and peaked T waves. This represents ischaemia Grade 1. (b) The collateral circulation supplying the LAD territory is evident. This provides partial protection, which explains the low grade of ischaemia. (c) The coronary angiogram of the same patient demonstrates an occluded left anterior descending coronary artery in its distal part (arrow).*

Pre-infarct ischaemias caused by acute and persistent obstruction of secondary arteries

Obstruction of the first diagonal artery, the first marginal circumflex artery, or the marginal right coronary artery induces a pre-infarct ischaemic pattern in the anterior wall. In particular, it is important to describe the isolated mid-anterior pre-infarct syndrome, which is characterized by a unique ECG pattern consisting of ST segment elevation with upright T waves in leads AVL and V2 (non-continuous leads) and ST segment depression accompanied by either inverted T waves in leads LIII and AVF (reciprocal changes) or upright T wave.[16] (see *Fig. 2.10*).

This pattern is produced by an obstructed first diagonal branch and is seen in three different clinical scenarios:

- as an initial manifestation of anterior pre-infarct syndrome involving the left anterior descending coronary artery;
- in isolated spontaneous obstruction of the diagonal branch; and
- in side-branch occlusion of the diagonal artery during angioplasty of the left anterior descending coronary artery.

The diagnosis is often overlooked during echocardiography, and therefore it is important to perform sestamibi scintigraphy to detect the infarct.

PRE-INFARCT ISCHAEMIAS OF THE POSTEROINFERIOR WALL

THE ECG AND CORONARY ANATOMY

In contrast to the anterior wall pre-infarction, in which the anterior wall is subtended almost exclusively by the LAD, in posteroinferior pre-infarction the posterior and inferior walls of the left ventricle are subtended by one of the two coronary arteries—right or circumflex—either predominantly by one, or by both (in which case they are said to be co-dominant).

The posterolateral area is usually nourished by the circumflex artery, but it may also be supplied by a dominant right coronary artery. The right ventricle is supplied almost exclusively by the right coronary artery and its branches. The size and interrelationship between the two circulatory systems (right and left) accounts for a great variety of ECG patterns in pre-infarction syndrome.

The right coronary artery may subtend opposing areas, such as the anterior wall and anteroparaseptal wall of the right ventricle and the posterior wall of the left ventricle. The left circumflex is also capable of supplying two opposing areas, such as the high anterior area (supplied by the first marginal) and the posteroinferior area subtended by the posterior descending artery. In 10% of the general population, the posterior descending artery arises from a major predominant circumflex artery.

PATHOPHYSIOLOGY

The ECG of a posteroinferior infarct may show different grades of ischaemia regardless of the dimen-

sions of the artery or the level of obstruction. The maximal changes are seen in lead LIII, since this lead records the inferior wall potentials. Lead LII records the posterolateral wall potentials, and lead AVF records the potentials between the inferior and the posterolateral wall (*Fig. 2.24*). Lead V1 records the potentials from the anterior and paraseptal wall of the right ventricle. When ischaemia in that area is caused by a proximal obstruction of the right coronary artery, the ST segment elevation in lead V1 is attenuated by the posterior opposite area or by lateral ST segment elevation.

In cases of isolated acute first right marginal arterial obstruction, the changes in leads V1 and V2 are not attenuated by the posterior injury; marked ST segment elevation in leads V1 and V3 may be recorded (*Fig. 2.25*).

THE ECG OF THE PRE-INFARCT ISCHAEMIAS OF THE POSTEROINFERIOR WALL

The ECG recorded during acute and continuing pain with upright T waves and ST segment elevation but without Q waves (or with non-significant Q waves) in the frontal leads (both bipolar and unipolar) reveals an acute and persistent obstruction of one of the epicardial arteries supplying the posteroinferior wall. Before the pre-infarction ECG patterns are analysed, it is necessary to recall that Q waves in the frontal plane area are very frequent in normal ECGs.

It is important to remember the patterns that can occur with varied ventricular rotations that may cause the appearance of Q waves in lead LIII. Three such patterns are dealt with here.

Pattern 1

The presence of Q waves in lead LIII and the presence of S waves in lead LI and in AVL is due to a counter-clockwise rotation of the frontal axis (*Fig. 2.26*). This syndrome is very frequent and is accompanied by other elements, such as an r' in AVR and a transition zone in the precordial leads with leftward deviation, causing S waves in all precordial leads (i.e. clockwise rotation). This pattern may mask the presence of pre-infarct ischaemia, especially when the ischaemia is of minor grade; in such cases the echocardiogram is a tool of great diagnostic help.

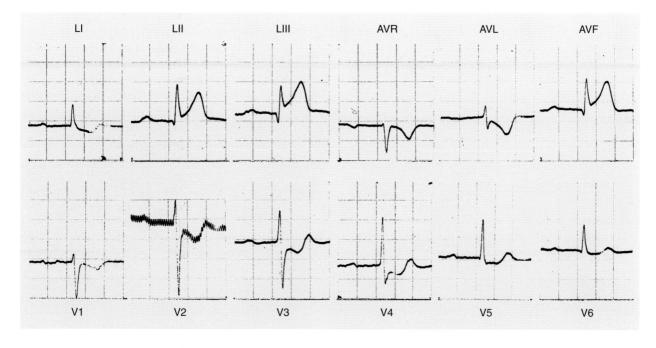

Figure 2.24 *Posteroinferior wall pre-infarct syndrome. After 30 minutes of symptoms, a qR pattern is noted in leads LII, LIII, and AVF with concave ST segment and peaked, tall T waves. There is a gradient in the severity of ECG changes from lead LIII through AVF and lastly in LII. Note that in AVL, an rS pattern is detected. A prominent S wave in AVL produces a posterior hemiblock-like pattern, representing non-uniform depolarization of the papillary muscles (see also Fig. 2.29).*

Pattern 2

This pattern is the ECG syndrome characterized by:

- the appearance of Q waves in leads LI, LII, and LIII (*Fig. 2.27*);
- deepening of the Q waves towards lead LIII;
- an initial r wave in AVR; and
- a transitional zone in precordial leads shifted towards the right between leads V1 and V2 (i.e. counter-clockwise rotation).

In these cases, the Q wave most probably does not represent necrosis. It is important therefore to identify this pattern (see *Fig. 2.27*).

Pattern 3

In ECGs with axis rotation to the right and downwards, qR waves in lead LIII are seen; these mask an inferior infarction of minor grades of ischaemia (*Fig. 2.28*). The various grades of ischaemia are also detected in pre-infarct ischaemia of the posteroinferior wall. The preinfarct ischaemias of the posteroinferior wall almost always culminate in infarction.

PRE-INFARCT GRADE 3 POSTEROINFERIOR ISCHAEMIAS

In most patients with posteroinferior ischaemia, the maximal grade of ischaemia is observed in lead LIII. The presence of Q waves in lead LIII in the very initial stages of the pre-infarct syndrome is the result of a unique mechanism. Owing to its location in the left ventricle, the early depolarization of the antero-superior papillary muscle produces a vector that is oriented upwards and to the left, while the early depolarization of the posteroinferior papillary muscle produces a vector that is oriented downwards and to the right. The algebraic sum of these vectors is seen in the initial vector of the frontal bipolar leads (*Fig. 2.29a*). The hemiblocks without infarction alter the sequence of these vectors. In anterosuperior

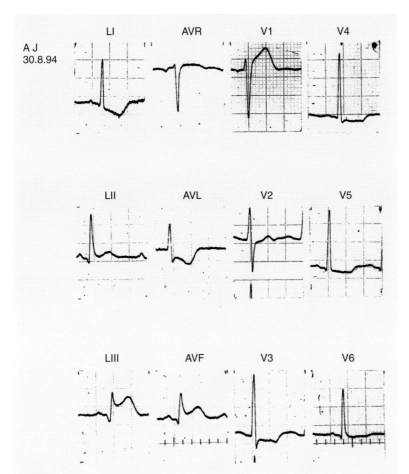

Figure 2.25 *An example of ST segment elevation in lead V1 which is proportional to LIII but is disproportionately greater than that in LII. This is due to the absence of severe ischaemia in the opposing wall to V1, manifested by LII, V5, and V6.*

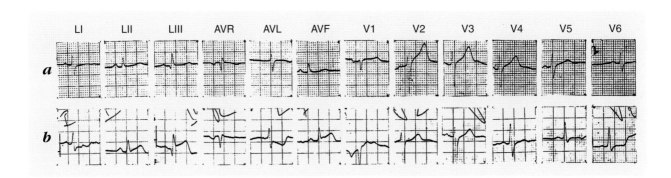

Figure 2.26 *(a) ECG with S1Q3 pattern (presence of S wave in lead LI and qR in lead LIII) in the steady-state. Note also the presence of r' in AVR and persistent S waves from V1 to V6. (b) Acute inferior wall pre-infarct syndrome in the same patient, with the previously noted q wave in lead LIII.*

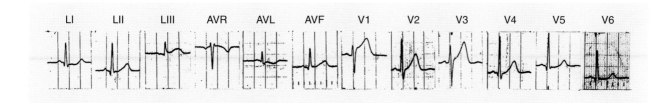

Figure 2.27 *Q1Q2Q3 syndrome. This is accompanied by an R wave in AVR and the absence of S waves in the left precordial leads. The Q waves in leads LII, LIII, and AVF do not indicate inferior wall infarction. The Q waves do not indicate inferior wall infarction. The ST-segment changes in lead L3, the ST-segment depression in lead AVL and the ST-segment elevation in lead V1 indicate an acute myocardial ischaemia in the right ventricle and inferior wall of the left ventricle.*

hemiblock, the posteroinferior papillary muscle depolarizes early in relation to the anterior muscle, thereby producing a positive initial vector in leads LII, LIII, and AVF (i.e. an r wave) and a negative vector in leads AVL and LI (i.e. a q wave) (*Fig. 2.29b*). Posteroinferior hemiblock induces an initial vector oriented upwards and to the left. This is seen by a q wave in lead LIII and the disappearance of the q wave in leads AVL and LI (*Fig. 2.29c*).

In the very early stages of pre-infarct ischaemia Grade 3, a q wave appears as a consequence of a delay in the early depolarization of the posterior papillary muscle relative to the anterosuperior muscle. This delay in the depolarization of the papillary muscles creates a vector oriented upwards and to the left. This results in a q wave in lead LIII, and the disappearance of the Q waves in leads LI and

AVL (see *Figs 2.24, 2.29d, 2,30a,b*). Again, this should not be mistaken for a reflection of necrosis.

This delay also causes the vectors that are depolarized later (after 40 seconds) to be oriented downwards and to the right. This is evident by increased R waves in lead LIII and increased S waves in AVL. This mechanism is responsible for the relatively more increased T waves and R waves in comparison with the ST segments (*Fig. 2.30*).

Anterosuperior hemiblocks with no acute ischaemia induce early depolarization of the posteroinferior papillary muscle, shifting the first vector downwards and to the right. This is reflected in the ECG as r' in leads LIII and AVF and q in leads LI and AVL. Therefore, most patients with pre-infarct syndrome and pre-existing anterosuperior hemiblock will have an ECG pattern entailing an r' wave in

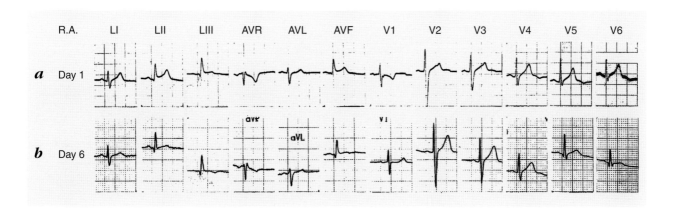

Figure 2.28 *(a) Inferior wall pre-infarct syndrome in a patient with qR pattern in lead LIII and rS pattern in AVF. Note the ST segment elevation in leads LII, LIII and AVF and the tall, peaked T waves in leads V4–V6. (b) Six days later, note that the qR and rS patterns have not changed, indicating that these changes are not reflective of the acute ischaemic event.*

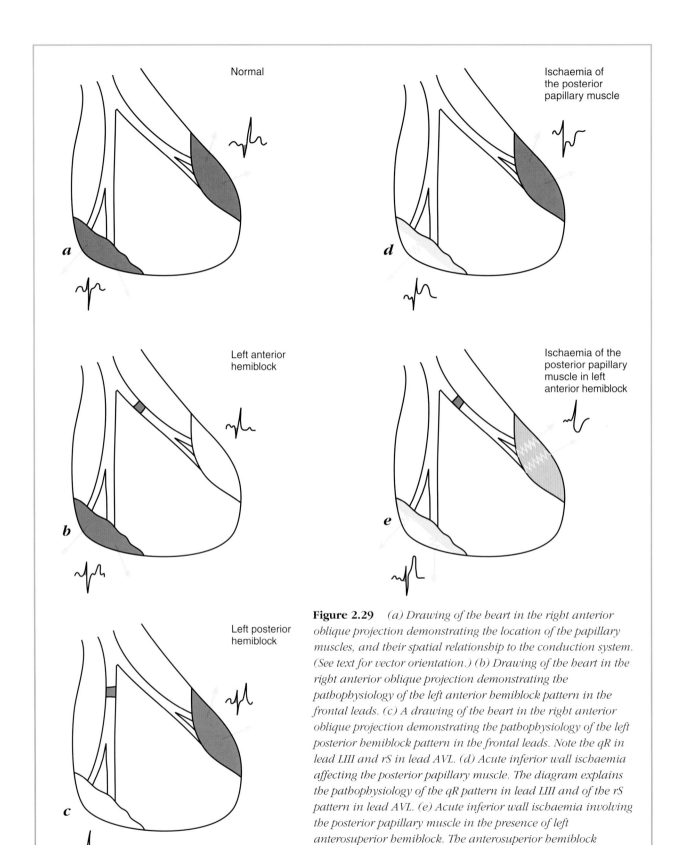

Normal

Ischaemia of
the posterior
papillary muscle

a

d

Left anterior
hemiblock

Ischaemia of the
posterior papillary
muscle in left
anterior hemiblock

b

e

Left posterior
hemiblock

c

Figure 2.29 *(a) Drawing of the heart in the right anterior oblique projection demonstrating the location of the papillary muscles, and their spatial relationship to the conduction system. (See text for vector orientation.) (b) Drawing of the heart in the right anterior oblique projection demonstrating the pathophysiology of the left anterior hemiblock pattern in the frontal leads. (c) A drawing of the heart in the right anterior oblique projection demonstrating the pathophysiology of the left posterior hemiblock pattern in the frontal leads. Note the qR in lead LIII and rS in lead AVL. (d) Acute inferior wall ischaemia affecting the posterior papillary muscle. The diagram explains the pathophysiology of the qR pattern in lead LIII and of the rS pattern in lead AVL. (e) Acute inferior wall ischaemia involving the posterior papillary muscle in the presence of left anterosuperior hemiblock. The anterosuperior hemiblock explains the absence of the q wave in lead LIII, and the persistence of the q wave in lead AVL.*

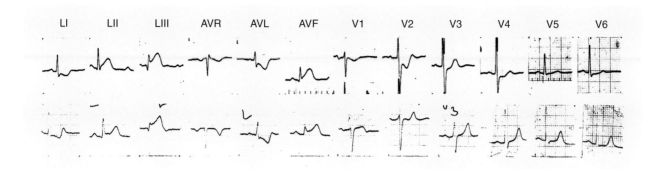

Figure 2.30 *Twelve-lead ECGs from two patients, demonstrating the presence of inferior wall ischaemia with the left posterior hemiblock-like pattern.*

leads LIII and AVF and persisting q wave in leads LI and AVL (*Fig. 2.31*). This mechanism is responsible for a proportional increase in the T waves, the ST segment, and the R waves.

As in anterior pre-infarction syndrome, the limb leads can also reveal several grades of ischaemia concomitantly. Ischaemia Grade 3 may be seen in only one lead (LIII), whereas ischaemia Grade 1 or Grade 2 may be seen in lead LII, and AVF shows an intermediate grade. Lead AVF records the posterior potentials of the area near the inferior wall while lead LII records the posterolateral potentials (far from lead LIII).[17] Therefore, in most inferior infarcts, lead LIII

shows the core of the ischaemia, AVF develops a grade equal to or less than that of lead LIII, and LII develops a grade equal to or less than that of AVF.

In posterior infarcts, the core of ischaemia will be seen in lead LII (*Fig. 2.32*). Most patients show marked changes in leads LIII, AVF, and LII; 20% show ECG changes in five leads (V5–V6 in addition to the three inferior leads) (*Fig. 2.33*) and 5% show ischaemia Grade 3 in all five leads. These have an extensive area at risk. Mortality among patients with ischaemia Grade 3 in five leads is around 12%, while mortality among patients with posteroinferior infarct is around 3–4%.[18]

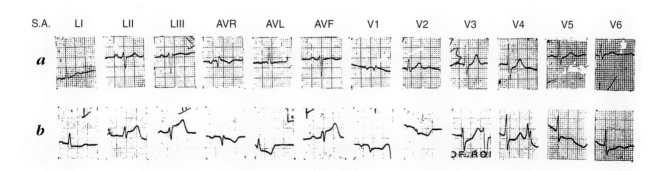

Figure 2.31 *(a) Twelve-lead ECG demonstrating the presence of left anterior hemiblock. (b) The same patient developed inferior wall ischaemia with the persistence of ECG abnormalities attributed to the conduction defect. Note that the first vector does not change in the acute pre-infarction syndrome.*

LI	LII	LIII	AVR	AVL	AVF	V1	V2	V3	V4	V5	V6

a

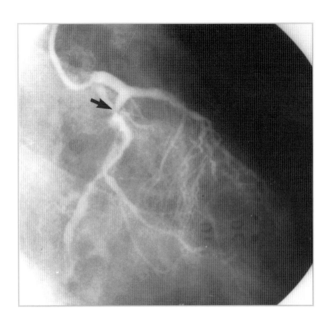

b

Figure 2.32 *(a) Pre-infarct syndrome with the maximal ST segment elevation in lead LII. These changes frequently are associated with lesions in the left circumflex coronary artery, as shown in (b). Coronary angiography revealed a severe stenosis in the proximal portion of the artery.*

PRE-INFARCT ISCHAEMIA GRADE 1

The pre-infarct syndrome shows peaked and tall T waves but no ST segment elevation. In general, this is not recognized as pre-infarct syndrome and is detected only in more advanced stages of infarction (*Fig. 2.34*). Ischaemia Grade 1 may appear in the core of the infarction or in the border zone such as leads LII, V5, and V6 of the inferior wall; most patients develop negative T waves in the border zone with ischaemia Grade 1.

ECG ANALYSIS IN POSTEROINFERIOR WALL PRE-INFARCT SYNDROMES

As for the anterior pre-infarction syndrome, the systematic analysis of the following parameters of the coronary anatomy should be considered in postero-inferior wall ischaemia:

- the culprit artery;
- the level of obstruction;
- the dimensions of the artery.

THE CULPRIT ARTERY

Unlike the situation in the anterior wall, where the predominant artery is the left anterior descending artery, the posteroinferior wall is supplied by two major epicardial arteries supplying and competing in the same ventricular wall: the right coronary artery and the circumflex artery. It is often difficult to identify the culprit artery.

When the right coronary artery is involved, the maximal sign of ischaemia is localized in lead LIII; LIII records the potentials of the inferior wall. Lead AVL shows the reciprocal changes of the inferior ischaemic vector (see *Figs 2.24, 2.25, 2.26b*). The inferior wall is supplied by the posterior descending artery, which in 80% of cases arises from the right coronary artery. This is why lead LIII generally

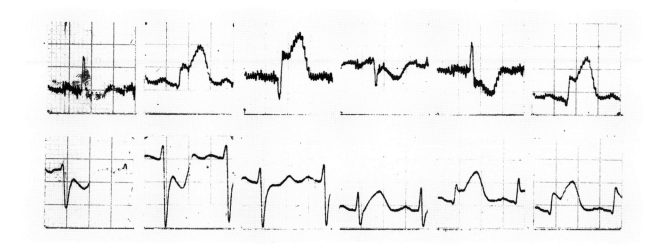

a

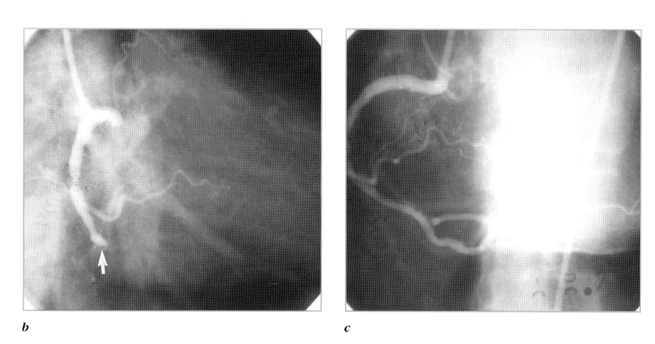

b   *c*

Figure 2.33   *(a) ST segment elevation in six leads associated with an acute obstruction of a predominant right coronary artery. The right coronary artery was suspected to be the culprit artery based on the presence of maximal ST segment elevation in lead LIII. The deep ST segment depression in the right precordial leads suggests a distal lesion in the right coronary artery, since the right ventricle was not involved (lack of ST segment elevation in lead V1). (b) This was confirmed by coronary angiography before angioplasty, which demonstrated an obstruction in the distal right coronary artery. The arrow points to the site of the obstruction. (c) After successful angioplasty, an especially predominant right coronary artery was detected.*

expresses ischaemias caused by the right coronary artery. The posterior, almost lateral, potentials are recorded by lead LII (*Figs 2.35, 2.36*). When the circumflex artery is involved, the maximal sign of ischaemia will be recorded in lead LII; it may reflect acute ischaemic processes of the lateral wall without

involvement of leads LIII or AVF (see *Fig. 2.6*). These changes may be accompanied by ST segment elevation in leads V5 and V6.[19]

Sometimes the ST segment has the same amplitude in leads LII and LIII. The level of the T waves may give an indication of where the core of ischaemia is

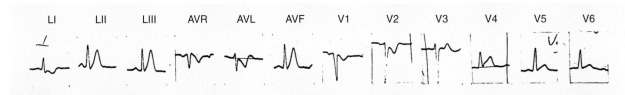

a

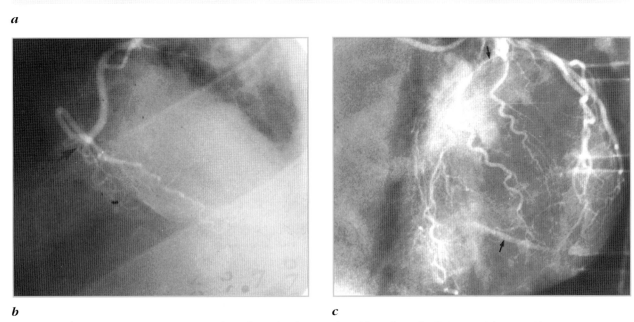

b   *c*

Figure 2.34 *(a) Ischaemia Grade 1 in the inferior leads, manifested by tall, peaked T waves. There is ST segment depression in leads LI, AVL, V2, and V3. This probably represents a reciprocal change to the inferior wall. (b) Coronary angiography was performed; this revealed an obstruction of the right coronary artery (b) with left-to-right collateral circulation (c), accounting for the low grade of ischaemia. The arrow in (b) points to the site of obstruction in the right coronary artery and in (c) the arrow points to the obstructed left anterior descending coronary artery and to the right posterior descending coronary artery which is nourished by collateral circulation.*

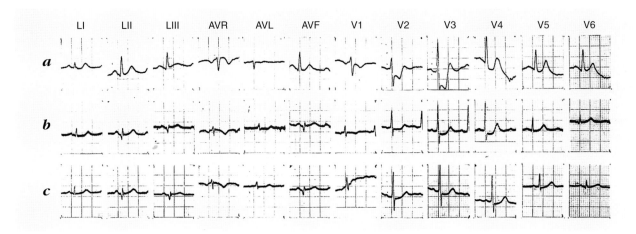

Figure 2.35 *These tracings demonstrate the importance of the T waves in identifying the culprit artery. In the examples shown, there is a similar degree of ST segment elevation in leads LII and LIII. However, in (a), the T waves in LII are of greater amplitude than those in lead LIII, suggesting that the culprit is the left circumflex. Moreover, the absence of ST segment depression in lead AVL indicates that the first marginal branch may be involved. Twenty-four hours later (b) the R wave became more prominent in leads V1–V2 and V5–V6. After 48 hours (c) these changes persisted.*

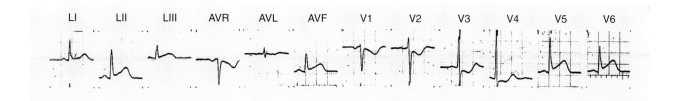

Figure 2.36 *Pre-infarct syndrome caused by acute occlusion of the left circumflex coronary artery. Note the presence of ST segment elevation in five leads (LII, LIII, AVF, V5, and V6), and the ST segment elevation, which is greater in LI than in AVL. The changes in AVL and LIII are attenuated because they face opposing walls with divergent injury vectors. Note also that the changes are more pronounced in lead LII than in LIII.*

(see *Fig. 2.40*). If the T waves are higher in lead LII it suggests that the culprit artery is the circumflex artery. If they are higher in lead LIII, the culprit artery will be the right coronary artery (see *Figs 2.30, 2.31*).

THE LEVEL OF OBSTRUCTION

The anterolateral wall of the right ventricle is subtended exclusively by the first marginal arteries of the right coronary artery. Right anterolateral wall involvement suggests acute obstruction localized to the proximal portion of the right coronary artery. The ECG will show inferior wall ischaemia, either with isoelectric ST segments or with elevated ST segments in leads V1, V3R, and V4R.

More distal obstructions (beyond the first marginal artery) will not compromise the right anterolateral wall, and the ST segment will be depressed in precordial leads with inverted T waves in leads V1, V2, and V3. This distal infarction may compromise the right posteroseptal wall without any ECG evidence.

When there is an isolated occlusion of the right marginal, considerable ST segment elevation may be observed in leads V1 and V2. These changes are prominent because there is no attenuation effect to counter the ST segment elevation in leads LII, V5, and V6 of the posterolateral wall (see *Figs 2.7, 2.25, 2.27*).

The circumflex artery supplies, by way of its marginal branch, the superior anterolateral wall. When the circumflex artery is occluded proximally, it will cause ST segment elevation with positive T waves in lead AVL and sometimes in lead LI (see *Figs 2.6, 2.35*). If the circumflex artery supplies the inferior wall of the left ventricle, the proximal acute obstruc-

tion will cause an 'attenuated pattern' because of the two vectors with opposing orientation. The ST segment in lead AVL will be slightly depressed and the T waves upright; the ST segment elevation in lead LIII will be also attenuated (see *Fig. 2.35*).

The ST segment depression in leads V1 and V2 will be very pronounced when the circumflex artery is obstructed, but this finding is not specific to that artery. The most sensitive sign for localizing the circumflex artery in posteroinferior wall preinfarction is the supremacy of lead LII in its grade of ischaemia (core of ischaemia) in relation to other leads: the core of ischaemia of the right coronary artery is localized in lead LIII (see *Fig. 2.33*). This fact will help to differentiate between distal ischaemias of these two arteries.

THE DIMENSIONS OF THE ARTERY

The length of the artery is determined by the number of leads involved in the process, thereby defining the area at risk. Pre-infarct ischaemia may involve only one lead or as many as five or six leads in the left frontal lateral leads (see *Fig. 2.33*). Obstruction of a small right coronary artery will involve only one lead, LIII.[20] If the occlusion of the small right coronary artery is in its initial portion, the right ventricle may also be involved, producing a right preponderant infarction. In this case, the ECG may manifest ST segment depression with inverted T waves maximally in lead V6 as a reciprocal sign of the injury vector oriented to the right (*Fig. 2.37a*). In distal obstructions of a small right coronary artery there may be signs of ischaemia in lead LIII.

One-lead ischaemia in LIII may also be caused by a distal obstruction of a branch of a right coronary

a

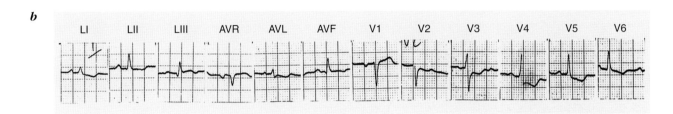

b

Figure 2.37 *(a) Single-lead ST segment elevation in inferior lead LIII. There is ST segment depression in AVL as a reciprocal change. Leads LII and AVF are not involved, implicating the right coronary artery as the culprit artery. Note the absence of changes in the precordial leads. (b) A similar pattern is seen, except for the presence of ST segment depression in left precordial leads. This pattern portends a poor prognosis.*

artery such as the right posterior descending artery (*Fig. 2.38*). In such cases, one of the most stable ECG signs is the appearance of ST segment depression and negative T waves in lead AVL.[21]

The obstruction of a small, distal circumflex artery will bring about a true posterior infarction, and the pre-infarct ischaemia diagnosis can be made by detecting reciprocal signs with ST segment depression and inverted T waves in leads V1, V2, and V3 (*Fig. 2.39*).[22]

The especially predominant right artery supplies the left inferior, posterior and lateral walls. Obstruction of the first part of the especially predominant right artery is a very dangerous condition, and it sometimes has a fatal outcome. In such cases the right precordial, posteroinferior, and lateral leads are involved. The most severe cases occur when the ischaemic process caused by the obstruction of the predominant right artery compromises the leads with ischaemia Grade 3 and the obstruction is proximal (i.e. acute obstruction can produce signs of ischaemia in the ECG lead). The final result in these cases is similar to an obstruction of the left main coronary artery.

Acute obstruction of the especially predominant right artery affects the inferior lateral portion of the left ventricle through the left lateral branch. The grades of ischaemia caused may vary from ischaemia Grade 1 to ischaemia Grade 3, and the effect on the ischaemic area is not always homogeneous throughout. In cases of left anterolateral and right ischaemia,

'attenuation' of the ST segment and T waves changes occur, since the same obstructed artery induces two vectors of opposing orientation. In cases of obstruction of the predominant right artery that causes ischaemia Grade 1 in the left lateral leads, it is difficult to diagnose the process at this stage; however the subsequent appearances of inverted negative T waves confirm the diagnosis of ischaemia Grade 1.

Acute distal obstruction of the especially predominant circumflex artery will induce ischaemia in multiple leads: LIII, LII, AVF, V5, and V6 (*Fig. 2.40*). In cases of proximal obstruction, leads LI and AVL may also be involved (see *Fig. 2.36*).

RECIPROCAL CHANGES IN PRE-INFARCT ISCHAEMIA

The presence or absence of reciprocal changes in posteroinferior infarcts is of great significance. There are three conditions in evolving inferoposterior infarction:[23]

- depression in all the precordial leads, more pronounced in leads V1 and V2 and decreasing toward leads V5 and V6 (see *Fig. 2.41a*);
- ST segment depression with negative T waves in leads V1–V3 (*Fig. 2.41b*);
- maximal ST segment depression and negative T waves in leads V4 and V6 (see *Fig. 2.41c*).

The precordial morphology may reflect involvement of the right ventricle. In spite of an ischaemic right

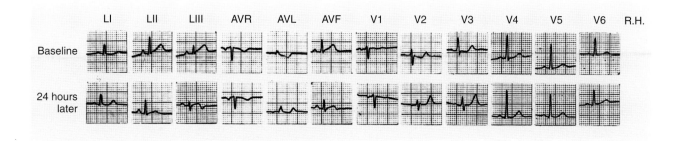

a

b

Figure 2.38   *(a) ECG tracings showing single-lead ST segment elevation in LIII, with reciprocal changes in lead AVL. (b) The coronary angiogram in the right anterior oblique position demonstrates an acute obstruction of the right posterior descending coronary artery (arrow).*

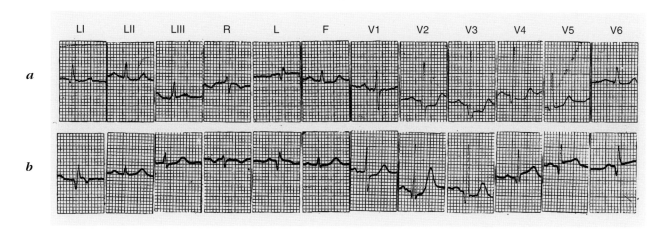

Figure 2.39   *(a) Posterior pre-infarct syndrome showing ST segment depression in leads V1–V3. (b) The subsequent ECG tracings revealed the evolution of posterolateral infarction.*

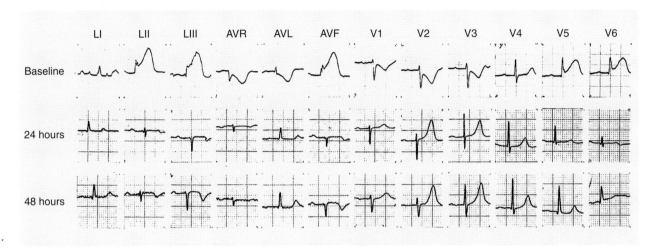

Figure 2.40 *Pre-infarct syndrome Grade 3 in leads LII, LIII, AVF, V5, and V6, caused by a distal occlusion of the left circumflex artery. Note the ST segment depression with inverted T waves in lead AVL. The T wave in LII is higher than the T wave in LIII.*

anterior wall, there is no ST segment elevation because of the 'attenuation' produced by the ischaemic vector opposite the posterior wall.

ST segment depression in leads V1 and V2 indicates extensive infarction of the posterior wall, in addition to infarction of the inferior wall. When lateral ischaemia is compounded by inferior ischaemia, ST segment depression in leads V1 and V2 is more marked.

ST segment depressions in leads V1–V3 are recipro-

cal changes, whereas ST segment depressions in leads V4 and V5 express the circumferential subendocardial ischaemia that is due to an increase in the LVEDP.[24]

Pronounced ST segment depression in leads V4–V6 is a severe prognostic sign. Inferior ischaemia, which is generally of low grade, produces an abrupt increase in the LVEDP, thereby inducing circumferential subendocardial ischaemia. Generally, patients with these ECG patterns suffer from severe coronary artery disease.

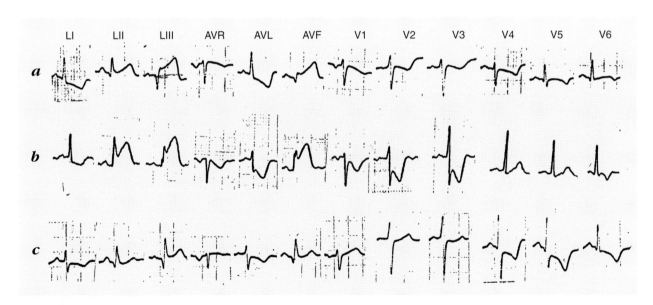

Figure 2.41 *Three types of reciprocal changes during inferoposterior wall infarction. (a) There is a progressive decrease in the degree of ST segment depression from V2 to V5. (b) Maximal precordial ST segment depression is seen in leads V2 and V3. (c) Maximal precordial ST segment depression is seen in leads V4–V6.*

REFERENCES

1. Fuster V, Baldinion LV, Baldinion JS, et al. The pathogenesis of coronary artery disease and the acute coronary syndrome. *N Eng J Med* 1986; **61:** 244–47.
2. Chesebro JH, Zoheligi P, Fuster V. Pathogenesis of thrombosis in unstable angina. *Am J Cardiol* 1991; **68:** B2–10.
3. Fowler NO. Preinfarction angina. *Circulation* 1971; **44:** 751–56.
4. Birnbaum Y, Sclarovsky S, Blum A, et al. Prognostic significance of the initial electrocardiographic pattern of patients with a first acute anterior wall infarction. *Chest* 1993; **103:** 1681–7.
5. Ben Gal T, Sclarovsky S, Herz I, et al. Importance of conal branch of the right coronary artery in patients with acute myocardial infarction: Electrocardiographic and angiographic correlation. *J Am Coll Cardiol* 1997; **29:** 506–11.
6. Birnbaum Y, Hasdai D, Sclarovsky S, et al. Acute myocardial infarction entailing ST segment elevation in lead AVL: Electrocardiographic differentiation among occlusion of the left anterior descending, first diagonal and first obtuse marginal coronary arteries. *Am Heart J* 1996; **131:** 38–42.
7. Birnbaum Y, Sclarovsky S, Solodky A, et al. Prediction of the level of left anterior coronary artery obstruction during acute anterior wall infarction by the admission electrocardiogram. *Am J Cardiol* 1993; **72:** 823–26.
8. Kurg SB, Douglas JS. Normal coronary artery in coronary arteriography and angioplasty. New York: McGraw Hill, 1985.
9. Tamura A, Kataoka H, Nagase K, et al. Clinical significance of lead inferior ST elevation during acute anterior wall infarction. *Br Heart J* 1995; **74:** 611–14.
10. Holland RR, Brooks H. The QRS complex during myocardial ischaemia: An experimental analysis of the porcine heart. *J Clin Invest* 1976; **57:** 541–50.
11. Vincent GM, Abildskor JA, Burgess MJ. Mechanism of ischaemic ST segment displacement: Evaluation of direct current recording. *Circulation* 1977; **56:** 556–9.
12. Silvester RH, Wagner NB, Wagner GS. Ventricular excitation during percutaneous transluminal angioplasty of the left anterior descending coronary artery. *Am J Cardiol* 1986; **62:** 1116–21.
13. Fuxiwara H, Asbraf M, Sato S, et al. Transmural cellular damage and blood flow distribution in early ischaemia in pig's heart. *Circ Res* 1992; **51:** 583–693.
14. Lavallee M, Cox D, Patrick T, et al. Salvage of myocardial function by coronary artery reperfusion, 1, 2 and 3 hours after occlusion of conscious dogs. *Circ Res* 1983; **58:** 235–47.
15. Sagie A, Sclarovsky S, Strasberg B, et al. Acute anterior myocardial infarction presenting with positive T wave and without ST shift: Electrocardiographic size of acute myocardial infarction. *Chest* 1989; **95:** 1211–15.
16. Sclarovsky S, Birnbaum Y, Solodky A, et al. Isolated midanterior myocardial infarction: a special electrocardiographic subtype of acute myocardial infarction with ST elevation in nonconsecutive leads and two different morphological types of ST depression. *Int J Cardiol* 1994; **46:** 37–47.
17. Shamroth L. *The Electrocardiology of Coronary Artery Disease.* 2nd edn. Oxford: Blackwell Science, 1984, p 53.
18. Herz I, Assali A, Adler Y, et al. New electrocardiographic criteria for predicting either the right or left circumflex artery as the culprit coronary artery in inferior wall acute myocardial infarction. *Am J Cardiol* 1997; **80:** 1343–5.
19. Assali A, Sclarovsky S, Herz I, et al. Comparison of patients with inferior wall acute myocardial infarction with versus without ST segment elevation in V5–6. *Am J Cardiol* 1998; **81:** 81–3.
20. Hasdai D, Yeshurun M, Birnbaum Y, Sclarovsky S, et al. Inferior wall acute myocardial infarction with one lead ST-segment elevation: Electrocardiographic distinction between a benign and a malignant clinical course. *Coronary Artery Disease* 1995; **6:** 875–81.
21. Birnbaum Y, Sclarovsky S, Mager A. ST segment depression in a VL: a sensitive marker for acute myocardial infarction. *European Heart J* 1993; **14:** 4–7.
22. Sclarovsky Y, Topaz O, Rechavia E. Ischemic ST segment depression in leads V2–V3 as the presenting electrocardiographic feature of posterolateral wall myocardial infarction. *Am Heart J* 1987; **113:** 1085–90.
23. Hasdai D, Sclarovsky S, Solodky A, et al. Prognostic significance of maximal precordial ST-segment depression in right (V1 to V3) versus left (V4 to V6) leads in patients with inferior wall acute myocardial infarction. *Am J Cardiol* 1994; **74:** 1081–84.
24. Hasdai D, Jabara R, Sclarovsky S, et al. Pathophysiology of precordial ST-segment depression in inferior wall acute myocardial infarction: an echocardiographic appraisal. *Cardiology* 1997; **88:** 361–66.

Chapter 3 Electrocardiography during reperfusion

SUMMARY

The ECG tracings obtained in the initial stages of reperfusion after pre-infarction syndrome are described in this chapter. In addition, the different scenarios during reperfusion are discussed and their identification using the ECG is described. The importance of differentiating between the normal patterns of reperfusion and re-ischaemia is stressed and explained.

INTRODUCTION

As discussed in Chapter 1, acute ischaemias are due to a sudden, transient obstruction, either mechanical or functional, of an epicardial artery. Reflow occurs spontaneously or following the use of vasodilatating drugs such as nitrates or calcium-channel blockers. The different patterns of myocardial reperfusion (phase II) in acute ischaemias have been discussed in Chapter 1.

One of the major aims of modern cardiology is to seek the most effective method of re-establishing circulation to the myocardial areas that are affected by persistent obstructions. The ECG is perhaps a unique non-invasive method of evaluating the reperfusion phenomenon. Moreover, systematic analysis of ECG patterns may reveal information not only about successful reperfusion, but also about the complications associated with reperfusion.

It is generally accepted that reperfusion of pre-infarct ischaemia occurs when the ST segment is elevated by more than half of its initial height.[1] This is 'the initial stage of reperfusion', but it does not indicate whether reperfusion has been complete or incomplete or whether it has been successful from the myocardial point of view. Complete reperfusion is a prolonged process that may last from a few hours to several days. In this chapter, only the initial stage of reperfusion will be analysed; the next stages will be dealt with in Chapter 4.

The ECG changes that occur during reperfusion depend on two factors:

- the coronary factor: how long the mechanical obstruction persists; and
- the myocardial factor: the effect of restoration of blood flow on the ischaemic muscle.

THE CORONARY FACTOR

Coronary angiography can give information about the grade of epicardial obstruction and the degree of reperfusion. However, it is well accepted that coronary angiography may not accurately describe myocardial blood flow.[2] The ECG, on the other hand, may offer insight into the myocardial blood flow and the status of the myocardium, including the metabolic changes that occur as a result of the washout of the catabolytes and electrolytes that will have produced ischaemic changes in the injured area.

THE MYOCARDIAL FACTOR

The grade of myocardial protection is of great importance for reperfusion. The greater the protection, the more the ability to withstand the ischaemic insult, thus enabling a greater time period to salvage the myocardium. As pointed out in Chapter 2, myocardial protection may be the result either of anatomical factors (such as collateral circulation or overlapping circulation from branches of two adjacent arteries) or of physiological factors (i.e. preconditioning).

CLINICAL STATES OF REPERFUSION

Taking into account both the coronary and myocardial factors, the ECG can show four clinical states of reperfusion (*Table 3.1*).

Table 3.1 Clinical states of reperfusion

Coronary	Myocardial
reperfusion	reperfusion (complete or incomplete)
reperfusion with no reflow	non-reperfusion
non-reperfusion	non-reperfusion
non-reperfusion	reperfusion (collateral circulation)

CORONARY AND MYOCARDIAL REPERFUSION

The serial ECG changes during reperfusion depend on the initial ECG pattern during the ischaemic episode. As described in Chapters 1 and 2, the ECG patterns can be divided into three grades of severity:

Ischaemia Grade 3

Ischaemia Grade 3 indicates that the ischaemic muscle lacks a protective mechanism. Hence the duration of obstruction must be very limited if reperfusion is to be effective at the myocardial level.

At this point, it is important to be aware of an ECG phenomenon that is frequently recognized because of early and repetitive recordings during the ischaemic process. The first ECG, obtained after 30 minutes to 1 hour from patients with acute ischaemia, often shows ischaemia Grade 3 (especially in the anterior wall). The ECG recorded 20–30 minutes later shows ischaemia Grade 2 or even a lesser grade of ischaemia (*Figs 3.1, 3.2*). These changes may represent spontaneous signs of reperfusion, anterograde or retrograde, sufficient enough to reduce ischaemia.

The first sign of reperfusion in patients with ischaemia Grade 3 type A is the reappearance of S waves; this phenomenon is observed especially in leads V2 and V3 (see Chapter 2 for additional details). The decrease in the amplitude of the ST segment together with a reduction in the amplitude of the T waves (to less than half of their initial level) is the most important sign of initial reperfusion, culminating in an ST segment of about 2–3 mm and T waves of about 5–6 mm in amplitude (*Figs 3.3, 3.4, 3.5*).

Ischaemia Grade 2

Ischaemia Grade 2 suggests that there is a major grade of protection in the affected myocardium.

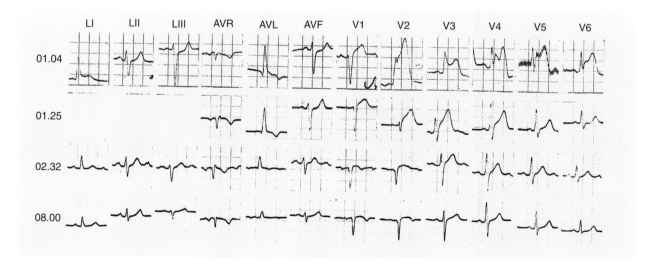

Figure 3.1 *ECG in the upper panel recorded in the Emergency Room obtained after 30 minutes of angina shows ischaemia Grade 3 from leads V2–V6. In the second panel, there is evidence to support spontaneous reperfusion–ischaemia Grade 2 from leads V2–V4 and ischaemia Grade 1 in leads V5 and V6. In the third panel, initial signs of reperfusion were evident. In the lower panel, an infarct pattern is noted with QS waves in lead V2.*

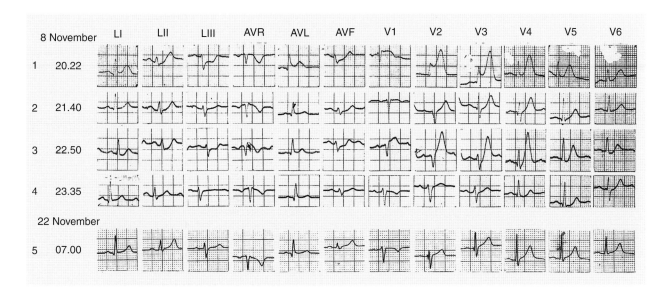

Figure 3.2 *ECG from a patient transferred from an internal medicine ward to the coronary care unit following 20 minutes of angina. Panel 1 shows ischaemia Grade 3 (type A) in leads V2 and V3. Panel 2 demonstrates evidence suggesting spontaneous reperfusion—an isoelectric ST segment with tall T waves. Panel 3 depicts re-ischaemia possibly involving the diagonal branch of the left anterior descending artery (ST segment elevation in leads AVL and V2, ST segment depression in lead LIII with inverted T waves, and ST segment depression with peaked, tall T waves in V3–V6). In panel 4, there is a marked decrease in the amplitude of the T wave, indicative of reperfusion. In panel 5, ECG characteristics of midanterior infarction can be seen.*

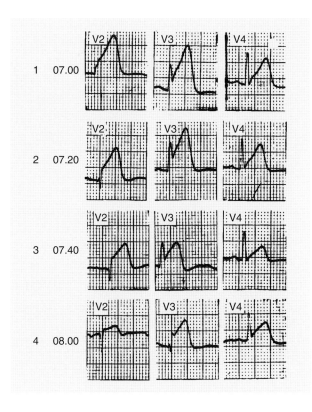

Figure 3.3 *Pre-infarct syndrome Grade 3 (type A) in leads V2 and V3. The first signs of ischaemia are evident in panel 1. In panel 2, the first sign of reperfusion is the reappearance of the S wave. There is no resolution of the ST segment or T wave. In panel 3, the ST segment elevation and T wave changes begin to resolve. This represents the first stage of reperfusion. The last panel shows the inverted T wave in lead V2, indicative of advanced reperfusion. This ECG sign is absent in the other leads.*

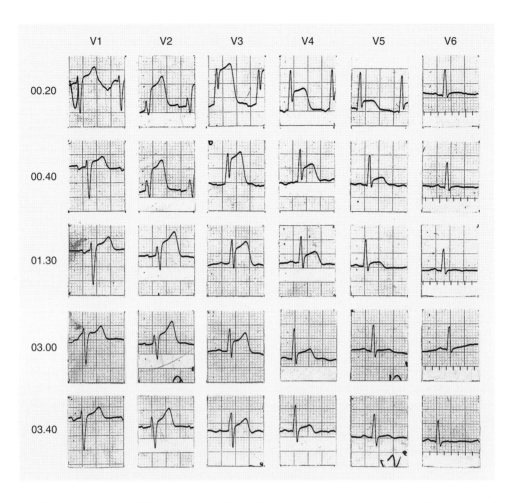

Figure 3.4 *Pre-infarction syndrome of the anterior wall. Serial ECG tracings from a patient with anterior wall ischaemia Grade 2 (type C). The first phase of reperfusion culminates when the ST segment elevation regresses to 2 mm in height and the T waves to 5 mm in height in involved leads.*

Therefore, effective reperfusion can be achieved even after prolonged obstruction. A frequently observed clinical pattern in the acute ischaemic syndrome with ischaemia Grade 2 has already been described (Chapter 2): the presence of ST segment elevation of 2–3 mm in leads V2 and V4, with T waves of 15–25 mm.

The most important sign of reperfusion in these cases is the progressive decrease in the size of T waves without any decrease of the ST segment (*Fig. 3.6*). Ischaemias of this type cause a significant accumulation of interstitial potassium ions in the epicardial area. Decrease of the T wave amplitude reflects a washout of potassium in the subepicardial area (*Figs 3.6, 3.7*).

Ischaemia with ST segment elevation and positive tall T waves may show an improvement in the elevation of the ST segment to 5–6 mm (when the initial elevation was 12–15 mm) and in the height of the T waves to 5–7 mm (when the initial height was 18–25 mm). In spite of the effective reperfusion according to the accepted criteria, this clinical condition may indicate a grave situation (*Fig. 3.8*).

The author defines the end of the first stage of reperfusion as being when the ST segment reaches 2–3 mm and the T waves reach 5–6 mm, regardless of the initial amplitude of the two parameters (see *Figs 3.4, 3.5*).

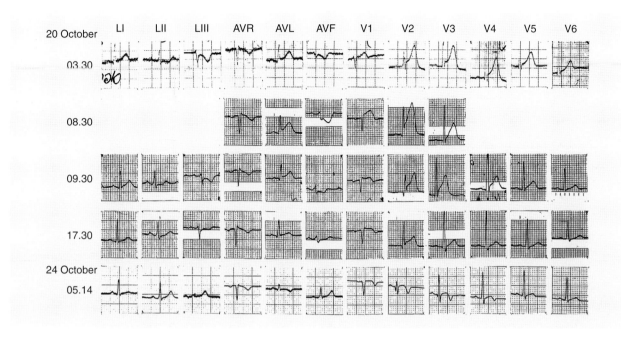

Figure 3.5 *Anterior wall pre-infarct syndrome with ischaemia Grade 2. This initial stage of reperfusion culminated in ST segment elevation of 2 mm and T wave amplitude of 5 mm. Initial reperfusion may be indicated by a reduction in the amplitude of the T waves rather than of the ST segments. In the bottom panel the isoelectric ST segment and inverted T waves indicate complete reperfusion.*

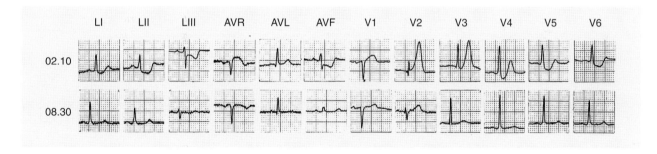

Figure 3.6 *Ischaemia Grade 1 in a typical tracing of a patient with an occluded diagonal branch. Note the tall and peaked T waves in leads V2 and V3. Reperfusion is indicated in this case by a reduction in the amplitude of the T waves rather than of the ST segment.*

Ischaemia Grade 1

In this type of ischaemia, effective reperfusion is supported by a decrease in the height of T waves toward the isoelectric line, especially in the border zone leads—leads V5 and V6 in anterior ischaemias and lead L2 in inferior ischaemias. These changes occur 12–48 hours after the reperfusion. Thus, there is a significant delay between reperfusion and the ECG manifestations of reperfusion among patients with this type of ischaemia (see *Fig. 3.6*).

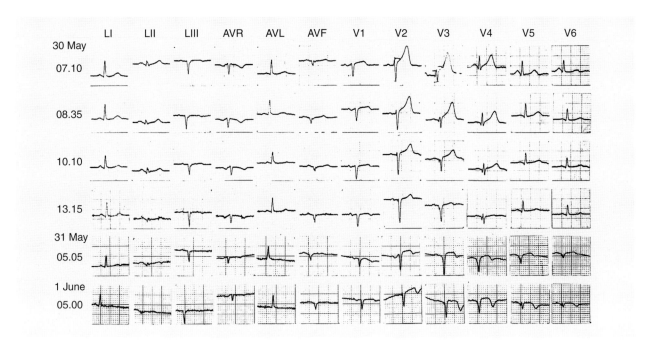

Figure 3.7 *Anterior wall pre-infarct syndrome. The ECG tracing demonstrates ischaemia Grade 2 (type A) in leads V2 and V3. The first stage of reperfusion is seen in panel 3. This manifests as a predominant reduction in the amplitude of the T waves. In these cases, there is no deepening of the S wave, but rather a cut-off of the R wave.*

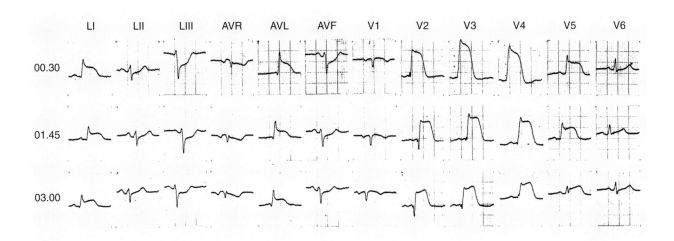

Figure 3.8 *Serial ECG tracings from a patient with ischaemia Grade 3 (type C) in leads V3–V5. Note that the amplitude of the ST segment and the T wave in leads V3 and V4 decrease but the original pattern persists. The bottom panel shows signs of reperfusion; however the ST segment elevation is about 5 mm in lead V2 and 7 mm in lead V3. This pattern predicts severe damage of the myocardium.*

CORONARY REPERFUSION–MYOCARDIAL NON-REPERFUSION (NO REFLOW)[3]

This phenomenon should be suspected when there is no further decrease in the ST segment toward the isoelectric level (beyond the initial 50% decrease). It is observed frequently in patients with ischaemia Grade 3 after 3 hours from the onset of symptoms, and in patients with ischaemia Grade 2 after 6 hours from the onset of symptoms. Coronary angiograms and ECG have to be recorded simultaneously in order to confirm this clinical picture. Coronary angiography shows signs of complete (TIMI 3) or incomplete (TIMI 2) restoration of epicardial flow, while the ECG will show no signs of metabolic restoration.

The clinical picture of reperfusion–non-reperfusion can also be detected in the catheterization laboratory when an occluded artery is treated with angioplasty, but in these cases the ECG still shows ST segment elevation and positive T waves.

In patients with ischaemia Grade 2, ECG signs of reperfusion are sometimes first seen 6 hours or more after the reperfusion of the artery (*Fig. 3.9*). A possible explanation for the difference between the grades of ischaemia is the extent of damage to the microcirculation, thereby preventing an effective washout of catabolytes and electrolytes accumulated during the ischaemia in the more severe types of ischaemia. The ischaemic process may also cause severe endothelial dysfunction at the microcirculation level in addition to the formation of platelet and neutrophilic microthrombi.[4] These processes may be most pronounced in patients with ischaemia Grade 3, less pronounced in patients with ischaemia Grade 2, and still less pronounced in patients with ischaemia Grade 1.

CORONARY NON-REPERFUSION–MYOCARDIAL NON-REPERFUSION

After administration of thrombolytic therapy or after unsuccessful angioplasty, the artery remains occluded. If the patient shows signs of myocardial protection (ischaemia Grade 1 or Grade 2), reperfusion may be effective up to 6–7 hours from the onset of symptoms. Unlike patients with the reperfusion–non-reperfusion picture (i.e. those with no reflow) discussed above, these patients who receive thrombolytic therapy may still achieve good reperfusion with rescue angioplasty, and this fact is of practical importance (*Figs 3.9, 3.10*).[5]

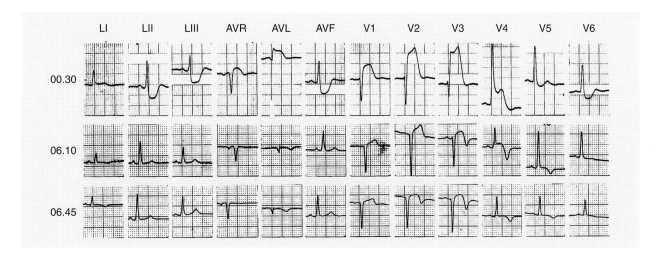

Figure 3.9 *Pre-infarct syndrome with ischaemia Grade 2 (type C). The first tracing was obtained 7 hours after the onset of pain. After angioplasty (rows 2 and 3), there are signs of reperfusion including a regression in the ST segment elevation and inverted T waves. These signs were most prominent in the last row.*

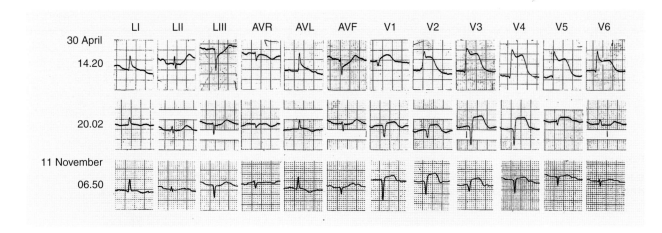

Figure 3.10 *Pre-infarct syndrome with ischaemia Grade 3 (type B), 3 hours after onset of pain. The ECG shows ST segment elevation of 5 mm in lead V4 and the T wave is of the same amplitude. Tracings obtained 12 days later still show significant ST segment elevation.*

CORONARY NON-REPERFUSION– MYOCARDIAL REPERFUSION

In this situation the artery is completely occluded (i.e. non-anterograde flow), but there are signs of myocardial reperfusion attributed to retrograde circulation or to perfusion from a neighbouring artery. The ECG shows peaked and tall T waves either with no ST segment elevation or with ST segment elevation of less than 2 mm in the precordial leads.[6] These patients suffer from chronic ischaemic conditions, because the critical obstruction of an artery has

allowed the evolution of collateral circulation (i.e. they have prepared collateral circulation). The thrombus occluding the culprit artery is usually very small (because the plaque burden is severe) and the ECG changes indicate ischaemia with a high grade of myocardial protection. The clinical picture of these patients depends on the grade of circulation evolved and the condition of the donor artery supplying the collateral circulation. If the donor artery is normal and the collateral circulation is effective, treatment of the culprit artery can be delayed (*Fig. 3.11*).

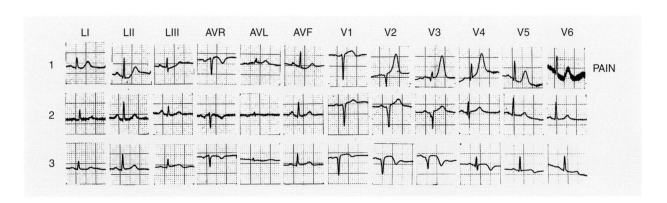

Figure 3.11 *Panel 1 (during pain) shows pre-infarction syndrome in the anterior wall with ischaemia Grade 1. Panel 2, recorded 12 hours later, shows Q wave reperfusion in leads V2 and V3 (first stage of reperfusion). Panel 3, recorded 3 days later, shows complete reperfusion.*

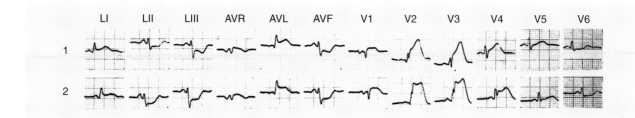

Figure 3.12 *Re-ischaemia after thrombolytic therapy. Panel 1 shows ischaemia Grade 2 pre-infarct syndrome. Note the involvement of leads AVL and LI. One hour after thrombolytic therapy there is re-elevation of the ST segment in leads V2 and V3 only and the QRS complex is consistent with ischaemia Grade 3 (panel 2). There are no changes, however, in the magnitude of the T waves.*

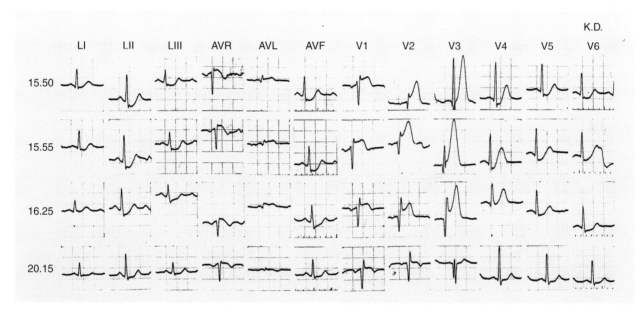

Figure 3.13 *Ischaemia Grade 2 in lead V2. After 5 minutes of thrombolytic therapy, there is partial resolution of the ST segment elevation. After 35 minutes of thrombolytic therapy there is re-elevation of the ST segment but the T waves are of lesser amplitude. This is probably an injury pattern rather than re-ischaemia, because the T waves have not grown in amplitude. Note the elevation of the ST segments and the reduced amplitude of the T waves in lead V3. Lead V3 is consistent with a QRS infarction. The last row depicts ECG signs of complete reperfusion.*

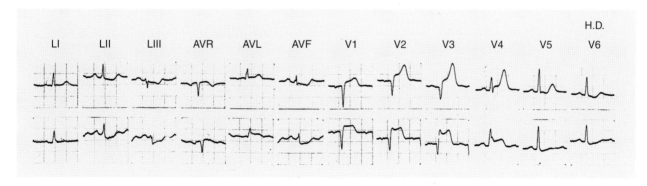

Figure 3.14 *Ischaemia Grade 2 in leads V2, V3 and V4. After 60 minutes of thrombolytic therapy there is re-elevation of the ST segment but the T waves are of lesser amplitude. This is probably an injury pattern rather than re-ischaemia, because the T waves have not increased in amplitude.*

ECG PATTERNS DURING REPERFUSION COMPLICATIONS

Scenarios associated with reperfusion recorded by the ECG are of two kinds:

- recurrent ischaemia; and
- arrhythmias.

In this chapter only the recurrent ischaemias are dealt with; arrhythmias are discussed in Chapter 6.

RECURRENT ISCHAEMIAS AFTER REPERFUSION

This phenomenon is indicated in the ECG by re-elevation of the ST segment during reperfusion. The ECG can demonstrate three types of re-ischaemia during the reperfusion process.

Type 1

This type is recognized by the transient re-elevation of the ST segment almost exclusively in leads with the maximal grade of ischaemia. This phenomenon is recorded in the early stage of the reperfusion process and always after the amplitude of the ST segment or the T waves has decreased. The re-elevation of the ST segment is not accompanied by an increase in the amplitude of the T wave. There is no increase in pain. These changes are usually transient (lasting only a few minutes). This type is commonly associated with a good prognosis. It can be explained by the mechanical effect of the abrupt onset of flow in the ischaemic area (*Figs 3.12, 3.13, 3.14, 3.15*).[7]

Type 2

This type of re-ischaemia is called phasic flow variations.[8] The ECG changes are more dramatic than those described above. They are seen in all the leads of the ischaemic area (core and border zones), and the grade of ischaemia that develops is Grade 3 regardless of the initial grade of ischaemia.[9] The maximal grade of ischaemia is observed in the leads facing the 'core of ischaemia', but advanced grades

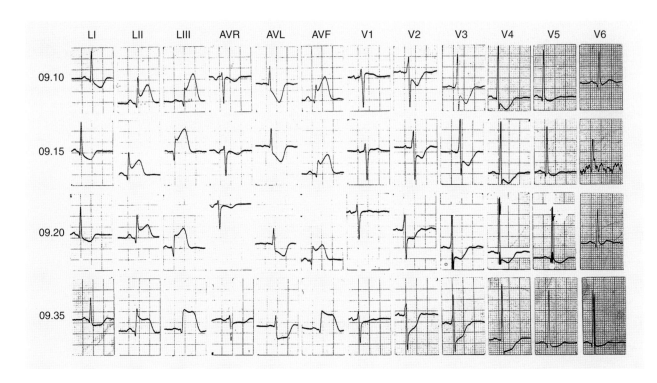

Figure 3.15 *A similar phenomenon to that described in Figs 3.12, 3.13 and 3.14 in a patient with inferior wall pre-infarct syndrome. Ten minutes after thrombolytic therapy there are signs of reperfusion. The last panel shows re-elevation of the ST segment and R waves but not the T waves.*

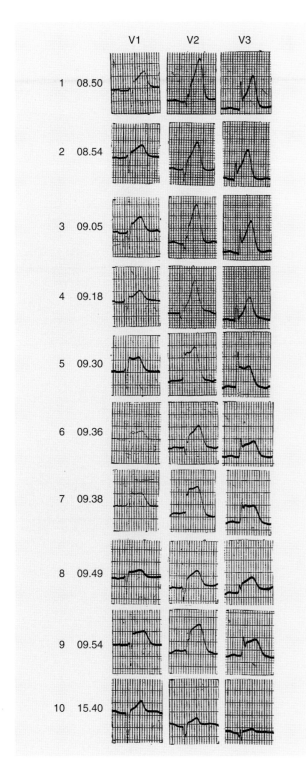

of ischaemia are also evident in the border zone leads (*Figs 3.16, 3.17*).

The underlying mechanism here is probably the release of platelet substances such as tromboxane B and serotonin, which affect the dysfunctional endothelium of the microcirculation. By causing the obstruction of the microcirculation, they eliminate the adenosine-dependent preconditioning effects, the collateral circulation that has developed, or the attenuated microcirculation of ischaemia in the border zone. These substances are responsible for repetitive re-ischaemias.[10]

The ECG changes may appear and disappear up to 10 times; they can appear within 20 minutes of the onset of treatment and last for up to a few hours. This phenomenon is observed in 30% of patients treated with thrombolysis and in 10% of patients who undergo spontaneous reperfusion. In such cases the treatment may include the administration of nitrates.

Type 3

The third ECG picture of re-ischaemia during reperfusion entails the appearance of ischaemia Grade 3 in leads V4, V5, and V6. This portends a poor prognosis. The apparent cause of this dramatic picture is myocardial haemorrhage or coronary embolism or both.[11] The maximal grade of ischaemia in leads V4, V5, and V6 is caused by an injury current that is oriented to the left, showing negative complexes in leads V2 and V3. These negative complexes may be due to a severe blockage of the septal depolarization (*Fig. 3.18*).

Figure 3.16 *ECG manifestations of cyclic flow variation after thrombolytic therapy. Panel 1 was obtained during the pre-infarct syndrome. Panel 2 shows signs of reperfusion (decrease in amplitude of the T waves and ST segment). Subsequently there were four episodes of re-elevation of the ST segment and T waves.*

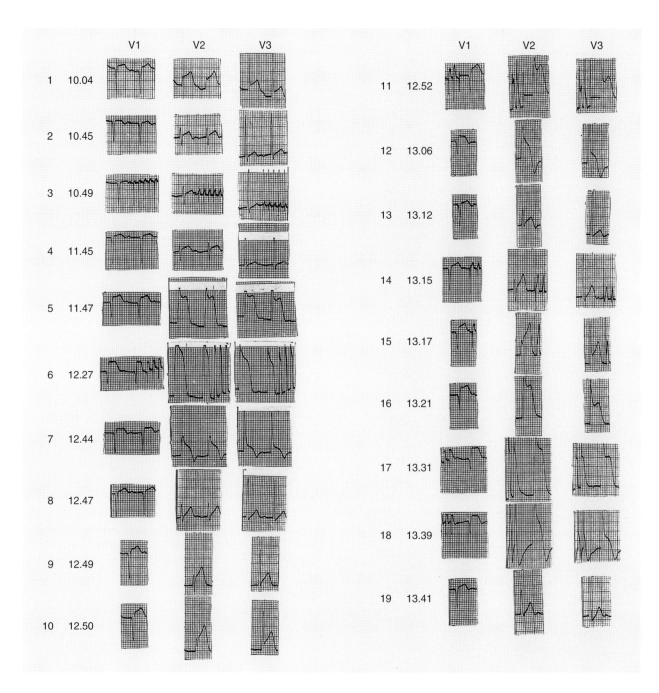

Figure 3.17 *Panel 1 shows ischaemia Grade 3. The fourth column indicates the first stage of reperfusion. One minute later (in panel 5) there is re-ischaemia with ischaemia Grade 3 pattern. At 12.52 and 13.17 additional episodes were noted.*

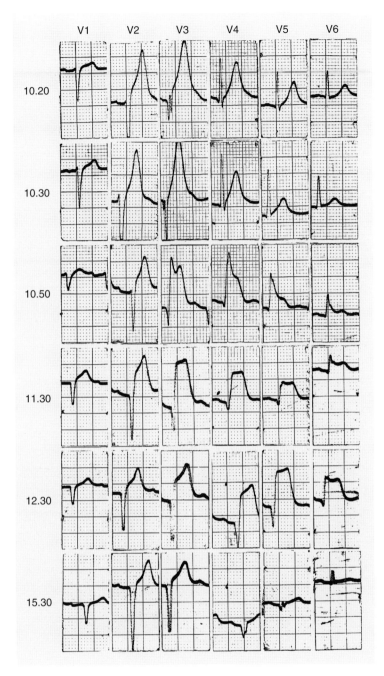

Figure 3.18 *Ischaemia Grade 2 in the anterior leads (panel 1). At 10.50 ischaemia Grade 3 appears, involving the lateral leads, which were relatively uninvolved beforehand. This patient died 24 hours later from cardiogenic shock.*

In summary, the typical ECG manifestation described in Table 3.1 is presented in Figure 3.19a–d.

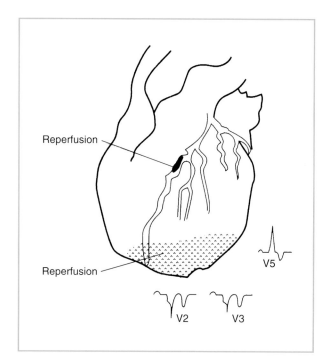

a

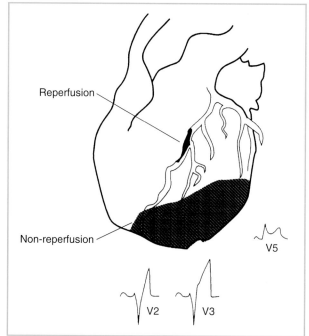

b

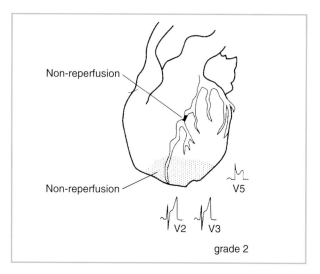

c1

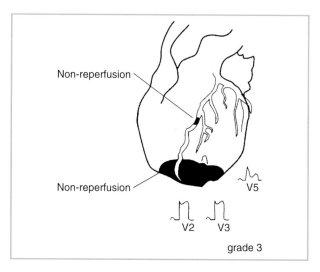

c2

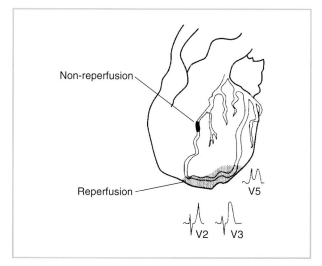

d1

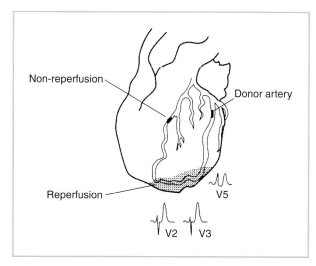

d2

Figure 3.19 *Typical ECG patterns during various conditions of perfusion. In (a), there is both coronary and myocardial reperfusion. The ECG pattern entails an isoelectric ST segment with inverted, peaked T waves. A QS wave of up to 10 mm in amplitude typically develops with a notch in the descending limb. In (b), there is only coronary reperfusion. The ECG pattern entails ST segment elevation with tall, upright T waves and a deep QS wave. In (c), there is no reperfusion of either the coronary artery nor of the myocardium. There is no Q wave. In Grade 2 (c1) (non-reperfusion), there is ST segment elevation with a positive T wave without distortion of the terminal portion of the QRS complex. In Grade 3 (c2) (non-reperfusion), there is distortion of the terminal portion of the QRS complex. In (d), there is only myocardial reperfusion. In (d1) there is collateral circulation resulting in the absence of ST segment elevation, although the T wave is tall and peaked. In (d2), the collateral circulation is attenuated because of disease in the donor artery. The ECG is identical to (d1), emphasising the need for coronary angiography to detect the difference between the two states.*

REFERENCES

1. Krucoff MV, Green CE, Satler LF, et al. Non invasive detection of coronary artery patency using continuous ST-segment monitoring. *Am J Cardiol* 1986; **57:** 916–23.
2. Lincoff AM, Topol EJ. Illusion of reperfusion. Does anyone achieve optimal reperfusion during acute myocardial infarction? *Circulation* 1993; **88:** 1361–74.
3. Kloner RA, Ganote CE, Jennigs RB. The "non reflow" phenomenon after temporary coronary occlusion in the dog. *Clin Invest* 1974; **54:** 1496–1508.
4. Kloner RA, et al. Ultrastructural evidence of microvascular damage and myocardial cell injury after coronary artery occlusion: which comes first? *Circulation* 1980; **62:** 945–53.
5. Mager A, Sclarovsky S, Herz I, et al. QRS distortion predicts no-reflow following emergency angioplasty in patients with anterior wall acute myocardial infarction. *Coronary Artery Dis* 1998; **9:** 199–205.
6. Sagie A, Sclarovsky S, Strasberg B, et al. Acute anterior wall myocardial infarction presenting with positive T wave and without ST shift. *Chest* 1989; **95:** 1211–15.
7. Kloner RA. Does reperfusion injury exist in human? *Am J Coll Cardiol* 1993; **21:** 537.
8. Ikeda H, Koga Y, Kowono K. Cyclic flow variation in a conscious dog model of coronary artery stenosis and endothelial injury correlated with acute ischaemic heart disease in human. *Am J Coll Cardiol* 1993; **21:** 1008–17.
9. Birnbaum Y, Sclarovsky S, Hasdai D, et al. ST segment reelevation after acute myocardial infarction: marked differences in the electrocardiographic pattern between early and late episodes. *Int J Cardiol* 1995; **48:** 49–57.
10. Galino P, Ashton JH, Gloss-Greenwald, A, et al. Mediation of reocclusion by thromboxene A₂ and serotonin after thrombolysis with TPA in a canine preparation of coronary thrombosis. *Circulation* 1988; **77:** 678–84.
11. Waller BF, Baum DA, Pinkerton CA, et al. Status of the myocardium and infarct related coronary artery in 19 necropsy patients with acute recanalization using pharmacological or mechanical or combined in reperfusion therapy. *J Am Coll Cardiol* 1987; **7:** 785.

Chapter 4   Acute myocardial infarction

SUMMARY

Various forms of ischaemia and infarction have been described in Chapters 1–3. Spontaneous or induced reperfusion often occurs in these states. It is important to identify the ECG changes associated with normal and abnormal reperfusion. In this chapter, the evolution of the ECG during complete and incomplete reperfusion is described. In addition, the author stresses the difference between transmural and subendocardial infarcts, and the ECG tracings obtained during reperfusion in these two types of infarct.

INTRODUCTION

Acute myocardial infarction is the final stage of the acute ischaemic syndrome. In Chapter 1, three ECG groups of acute ischaemias produced by a sudden occlusion of a coronary artery were discussed:

- acute regional transmural ischaemia;
- acute regional subendocardial ischaemia; and
- acute circumferential subendocardial ischaemia.

Each type of ischaemia may subsequently result in infarction, by way of the pre-infarct syndrome. In addition, each type will produce an infarction with distinct haemodynamic, ECG and prognostic characteristics.

In this chapter, ECG characteristics of these acute infarcts will be analysed.

ACUTE REGIONAL TRANSMURAL INFARCTION

Regional transmural pre-infarct syndrome may evolve towards myocardial infarction with or without Q waves developing in the ECG tracing. Whether infarction with or without Q waves evolves depends on two factors:

- the length of time that the thrombus obstructs the artery; and
- the capacity of the myocardium to develop protective mechanisms.

If the occlusion is promptly resolved, the lesion may be minimal (non-Q wave). The infarct process is implicated by ancillary biochemical tests (such as creatine kinase) or on ECG as an alteration of repolarization (inverted T waves) or a decrease in the size of R waves. Because the Q waves may appear only after 72 hours, the diagnosis of non-Q wave myocardial infarction should not be made until 4 days after the acute event.

ACUTE REGIONAL TRANSMURAL INFARCTION WITH Q WAVES

The pre-infarct syndrome may evolve toward a Q wave infarct in three circumstances:

- complete epicardial reperfusion;
- incomplete epicardial reperfusion;
- myocardial non-reperfusion.

The ECG may reflect each of these circumstances. In Chapter 3, it was mentioned that the accepted ECG sign of reperfusion is a 50% decrease in the amplitude of the ST segments and the T waves. The decrease in the ST segments to 2–3 mm and in the T waves to 6–7 mm is the first stage of reperfusion. The reperfusion process may stop at this stage and not evolve to more advanced stages (*Fig. 4.1*). Serial tracings are needed to recognize subsequent signs of effective reperfusion at the coronary and myocardial level. To understand the ECG signs of reperfusion it

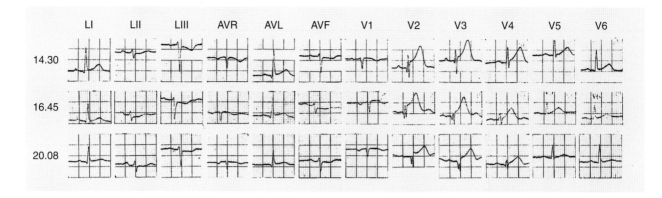

Figure 4.1 *Progressive disappearance of the R waves in the anterior leads in a patient with anterior infarction and ischaemia Grade 2. Although there are signs of reperfusion, the patient did not progress beyond the first stage of reperfusion—that is, he did not develop isoelectric ST segments and the T waves remained upright. Note that T1 slopes upward whereas T2 slopes downward. This represents incomplete reperfusion.*

is important to analyse the T waves thoroughly. The T waves are composed of two limbs, T1 and T2.[1]

The ECG can recognize three stages of effective reperfusion (*Fig. 4.2*):

- inversion of the T2 waves while T1 is still upright and elevated along with the ST segment;
- inversion of the two limbs of the T waves, with the peak being inverted and beneath the isoelectric line. The ST segment still remains elevated above the isoelectric line; and
- inversion of the T waves with an isoelectric ST segment.

While the ST segment and the T waves evolve towards complete reperfusion, a q wave progressively appears. In anterior infarcts, q waves appear principally in the leads with maximal grade of ischaemia in the 'core of the infarction' (leads V2 and V3). It is important to distinguish between q waves that represent reperfusion from those that represent non-reperfusion. The typical q wave associated with reperfusion is characterized by a qS of less than 10–12 mm in leads V2 and V3 and by the existence of a 'notch wave' in the descending limb of the q wave.

Thus, complete reperfusion is supported by the presence of q waves as described above, isoelectric ST segments, and inverted T waves (see *Fig. 4.2*). The inversion of the T waves represents complete electrophysiological reperfusion. This inverted T wave is a recording of the subendocardial QT segment, which is shorter than the epicardial QT

segment.[2] In contrast, during acute ischaemia the T wave is tall and peaked because the epicardial QT segment is shorter owing to the hyperpolarization phenomenon of the epicardial layer.[3] When the metabolites of ischaemia are washed out, the epicardial QT segment becomes prolonged.

In anterior infarcts, this phenomenon is seen in leads V2 and V3 (*Fig. 4.3*). In lead V4 the q wave appears later; in leads V5 and V6 it may appear much later (after 24–48 hours). These represent more protected areas, which can delay the appearance of the q wave (*Fig. 4.4*).

When reperfusion q waves develop in the absence of an isoelectric ST segment, this represents different pathophysiologies and prognosis. The development of a reperfusion q wave with a slightly elevated ST segment will commonly result in the gradual re-elevation of the ST segment and pseudonormalization of the T waves, usually seen after 4–5 days (*Fig. 4.5*; see also Chapter 5).

In addition, reperfusion q waves with ST segment depression suggest extensive coronary artery disease, causing an increase in the end-diastolic pressure and thus leading to subendocardial injury. The pattern of reperfusion in patients with ischaemia Grade 3 evolves from QR to qS (*Fig. 4.6*). In ischaemia Grade 2, the R waves diminish progressively during reperfusion, culminating in the QS pattern (see *Figs 4.1, 4.4, 4.5*).

Pre-infarct ischaemia Grade 2 with moderate ST segment elevation (2–3 mm) and tall T waves (15–25 mm) will show a regional subendocardial qRS

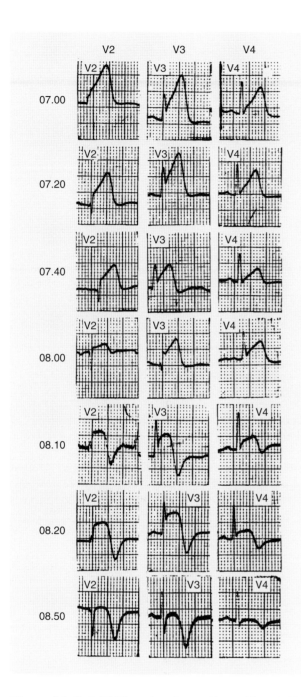

Figure 4.2 *Serial ECG tracings in a patient with anterior wall pre-infarct syndrome and ischaemia Grade 3 (type A) in lead V2, and ischaemia Grade 2 in leads V3 and V4. Until 08.00 the ECG evolved to the first stage of reperfusion. Note that before the resolution of the ST segment elevation in lead V2, there is a gradual reappearance of the S wave. At 08.10 and thereafter the second and third stages of reperfusion became evident. The bottom panel shows a reperfusion q wave in lead V2, characterized by a QS of 8 mm and a notch in the ascending limb of the QS, as well as an isoelectric ST segment and a deeply inverted T wave.*

pattern. This is frequently seen in lead V4 and occasionally in leads V3 or V5 (*Fig. 4.7*). In pre-infarction syndrome with ischaemia Grade 2, the reperfusion signs can be delayed over 24 hours; this phenomenon is called the 'stuck pattern'; it will rarely be seen in a higher degree of ischaemia Grade 3 (*Fig. 4.8*).

Pre-infarct ischaemia Grade 1 typically evolves slowly—many hours may pass until changes in the morphology become evident. This phenomenon is also observed in anterior ischaemia Grade 1 in leads V5 and V6 (see *Fig. 4.4*).

In the inferior wall, reperfusion may be seen only in the ST segment and the T waves while the QR retains its initial morphology (*Fig. 4.9*). This is because of the lack of homogeneity of depolarization between the papillary muscles. The QS pattern may appear a few days later or the QR wave may remain unchanged; the unchanged QR pattern almost always suggests a complete obstruction of the right coronary artery with collateral circulation.

In contrast to anterior wall infarcts, in inferior wall infarcts with q wave reperfusion, the depth of the qS complex is of no diagnostic or prognostic significance and there is no 'notch wave'. Ischaemia Grade 2 or Grade 1 presenting in lead LII will evolve toward infarction within 24–72 hours; the more advanced the ischaemia in this lead the sooner reperfusion q waves will appear. Thus, a patient with ischaemia Grade 3 and reperfusion will develop q waves rapidly (*Fig. 4.10*). Infarction with q wave reperfusion may evolve rapidly (within 2–4 hours) towards the final stage (QS waves, isoelectric ST segment, and negative T waves) (see *Fig. 4.10*) or very slowly (within 12–72 hours) (*Fig. 4.11*).

Reperfusion q waves are frequently seen immediately after successful angioplasty in patients with acute total obstruction and effective coronary and myocardial reperfusion (*Fig. 4.12*).

The ECG recording is therefore of crucial importance in evaluating the effect of the mechanical reperfusion.

NON-REPERFUSION q WAVE

In contrast to the reperfusion q wave, the non-reperfusion q wave is not accompanied by other ECG signs of reperfusion, and the qS wave gradually increases in amplitude. The qS is also different from that associated with reperfusion (*Fig. 4.13*):[2]

- the QS is deep—between 15 mm and 25 mm;
- the descending limb of the Q wave is not notched.

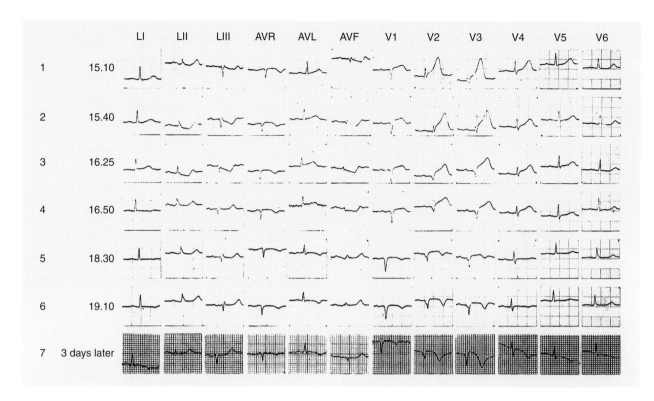

Figure 4.3 *An example of reperfusion q waves. The first tracing depicts anterior pre-infarct syndrome with ischaemia Grade 2. Subsequent tracings demonstrate a progressive disappearance of the R wave, concomitantly with the regression of the ST segment elevation and peaked T waves. Panel 4, showing the tracing obtained 100 minutes after the initial ECG, represents the first stage of reperfusion. Panel 5 exhibits the second phase of reperfusion—inverted T waves in leads V2 and V3 with ST segment elevation. Panel 7 depicts the ECG tracing obtained 3 days later; reperfusion q waves are evident along with the isoelectric ST segment and the deep inverted T waves. Note that the leads with the least severity of ischaemia (leads V5 and V6) are the last to manifest inverted T waves.*

In anterior infarcts, the depth depends on the electrical potentials caused by the reciprocal wall; these potentials are brought about by hypercontractility of the posterior wall, which is caused by deep injury (from the epicardium to the endocardium) of the anterior myocardium. Some of these cases evolve toward the pattern of incomplete reperfusion (deep qS, elevated ST segment, and T1 and negative T2 after about 72 hours). The elevated ST segment and the permanent tall and peaked T waves are due to a completely or incompletely non-reperfused artery in the presence of a very damaged microcirculation, which does not permit the washout of the substances that affect the ischaemic myocardium. Angio-plasty may produce TIMI 3, but the ECG continues to show the inability of the microcirculation to wash out the waste products.

ACUTE REGIONAL SUBENDOCARDIAL INFARCTION

If regional subendocardial ischaemia (shown on the ECG by ST segment depression with positive, peaked, and tall T waves) persists long enough, it will evolve towards the initial stage of regional subendocardial infarction. The subendocardial injury

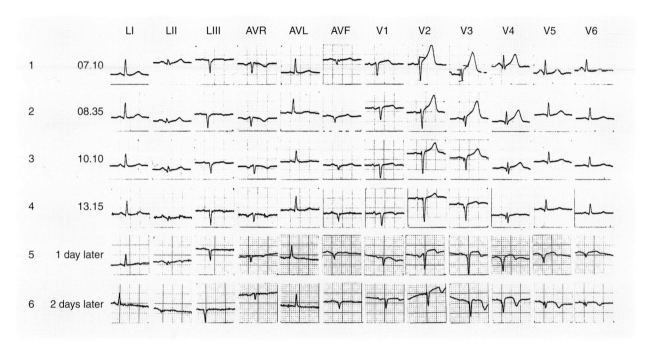

Figure 4.4 *Panel 1 depicts anterior pre-infarct syndrome with ischaemia Grade 2 (type A) in lead V2. Tracings during the next 3 hours demonstrate a gradual decrease in the amplitude of the R wave in leads V2–V4. Note the marked decrease in the magnitude of the T waves, and less so the ST segment. Panel 4, obtained 6 hours after the first ECG, illustrates the first stage of reperfusion with reperfusion q waves and mild ST segment elevation. In lead V3, there is an inversion of the T2 limb. Panel 5 shows the ECG the following day; this is the second stage of reperfusion characterized by inverted T waves and persistent ST segment elevation. Panel 5, obtained 2 days later, shows signs of complete reperfusion—an isoelectric ST segment and deeply inverted T waves. Note the late appearance of q waves in leads V5 and V6, which were only mildly ischaemic during the acute episode (ischaemia Grade 1). As explained in the text, the more severe the ischaemia, the sooner the appearance of q waves.*

depends on the intensity of the ischaemia. The regional subendocardial ischaemia evolves as an ECG cascade:

- Grade 1: the T waves become positive and there is a slight depression of ST segment;
- Grade 2: significant ST segment depression develops and the T waves are peaked and tall;
- Grade 3: the terminal portion of the QRS complex becomes distorted (S waves disappear, Q waves appear transiently and the ST segment is isoelectric with peaked and tall T waves) (see Chapter 1).

The time taken to reach the initial pattern of

infarction depends on the grade of subendocardial ischaemia developed.

Regional anterior subendocardial infarcts are probably caused by an acute, critical, and incomplete obstruction of the left anterior descending artery.[4] It is rare to see regional inferior subendocardial infarcts. It is not uncommon for the regional subendocardial ischaemias to evolve towards regional transmural infarction in the same ECG leads as those affected in subendocardial infarcts (because there is a complete obstruction of the left anterior descending artery by the thrombus).

As stressed in Chapter 3, ST segment depression in the precordial leads is in fact evidence of ST segment elevation (injury pattern) produced in the

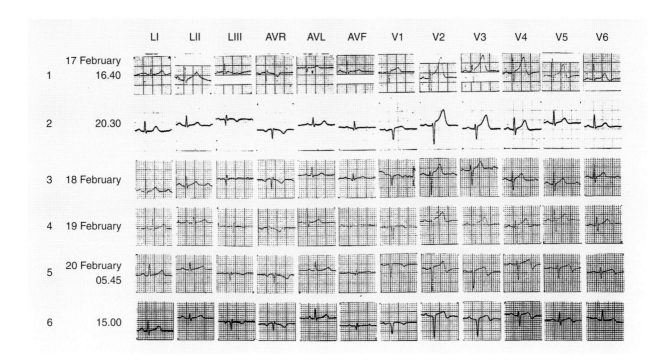

Figure 4.5 *An example of reperfusion after anterior infarction, with persistent ST segment elevation and inverted T waves several days later. As shown in panel 4, the patient achieved the first stage of reperfusion only after several days. Panel 5, obtained 4 days later, represents the second stage of reperfusion in leads V2–V6—inverted T2 wave but T1 and ST segment are still elevated. Panel 6 shows that, 12 hours later, this pattern persists. This represents incomplete reperfusion. As discussed in Chapter 5, these patterns often show subsequent pseudonormalization of the T waves, which represents infarct expansion rather than infarct extension or re-ischaemia.*

subendocardial layer as recorded by intracavitary potentials.[5] Extensive research on the physiology of the subendocardial layer (in the experimental laboratory) has revealed important information for interpreting the phenomenon of regional subendocardial infarction. When an incomplete, proximal stenosis produces hypoperfusion, the ischaemia usually occurs in the subendocardium. Recently it has been demonstrated that, regardless of differences in blood flow between the endocardium and epicardium, the endocardium may have an inherently greater susceptibility to ischaemic injury than the subepicardium.[6]

Stress and consequently oxygen demand are greater in the inner than the outer layer of left ventricular wall. Therefore the inner layer has a higher concentration of glycolytic enzymes,[7] greater oxygen

extraction,[8] and faster lactate production during ischaemia.[9] The data suggest a higher metabolic level in the endocardium than in other layers of the myocardium.

Q WAVE APPEARANCE IN REGIONAL SUBENDOCARDIAL INFARCTION

Regional subendocardial infarction may be expressed by a tiny Q wave followed by a normal RS complex (*Fig. 4.14*), or it may appear with an 'embryonic R' in the descending limb of the Q waves in leads V3 and V4 (*Fig. 4.15*).

Necrosis of the regional subendocardial layer is manifested by a Q wave, owing to 'unopposed forces' (that is the disappearance of the 'cancellation

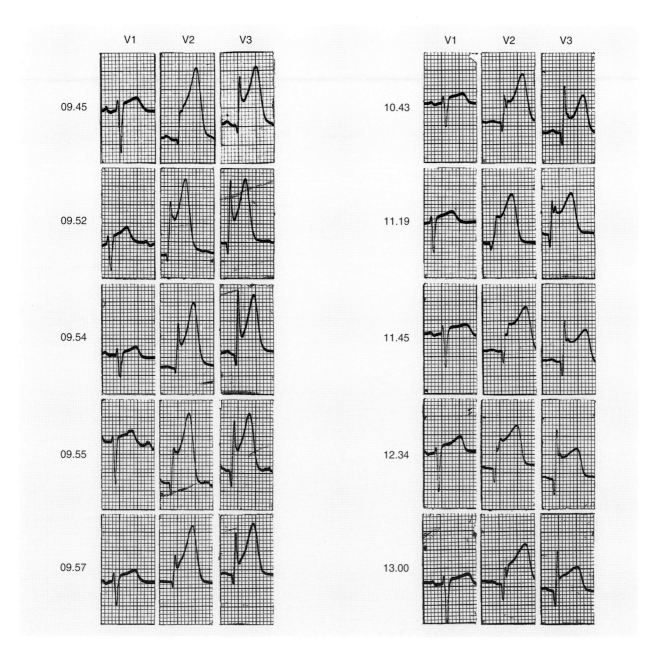

Figure 4.6 *Anterior wall pre-infarct syndrome with ischaemia Grade 3 (type A). Over more than 4 hours, there is a gradual decrease in the ST segment elevation by more than 50%, with a similar trend for the T wave. However, the ST segment is still significantly elevated (6 mm) as is the T wave (11 mm). Note the progressive appearance of the q wave and the development of qR. These patients often have a poor prognosis because of ineffective reperfusion (i.e. they had not achieved the first stage of reperfusion).*

phenomenon' in that area). Durrer confirmed experimentally that, in regional subendocardial infarcts, the tiny Q-wave precedes the RS complex.[10] This small Q wave is due to a limited lesion in the subendocardial layer. The myocardium above the lesion is depolarized by tangential vectors (*Fig. 4.16*). As the lesion penetrates deeper into the myocardium, the Q waves become more pronounced and the R waves become smaller (*Fig. 4.17*). The last grade of this type of lesion is the appearance of an 'embryonic R'

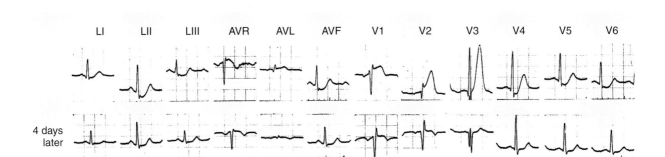

Figure 4.7 *Acute anterior wall pre-infarct syndrome. In leads V2 and V3 there is ischaemia Grade 2 (type A). Note the tall and peaked T waves (20 mm from the isoelectric line). Four days later, there is a significant decrease in the amplitude of the T wave, and in lead V3 there is a QRS pattern infarction.*

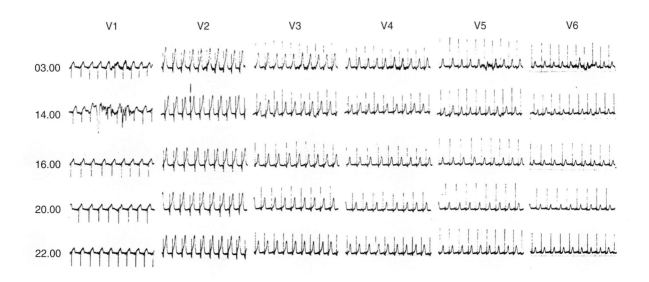

Figure 4.8 *Continuous 6-channel ECG recordings at 5 mm/sec over 18 hours. Note the ischaemia Grade 2 (type A) pattern in V2—V4. There is ST segment elevation of 2 mm in V2 and V3. After 18 hours there is no change in this pattern (stuck pattern).*

wave in the descending limb of a deep Q wave.[10] The qRS wave may also evolve from a regional trans-mural ischaemia in which the necrotic process has stopped in the early stages (see *Fig. 4.7*).

ACUTE CIRCUMFERENTIAL ISCHAEMIA EVOLVING TO ACUTE MYOCARDIAL INFARCTION

Circumferential ischaemias are recognized by the sudden appearance of ST segment depression with negative T waves, maximal in leads V4 and V5,

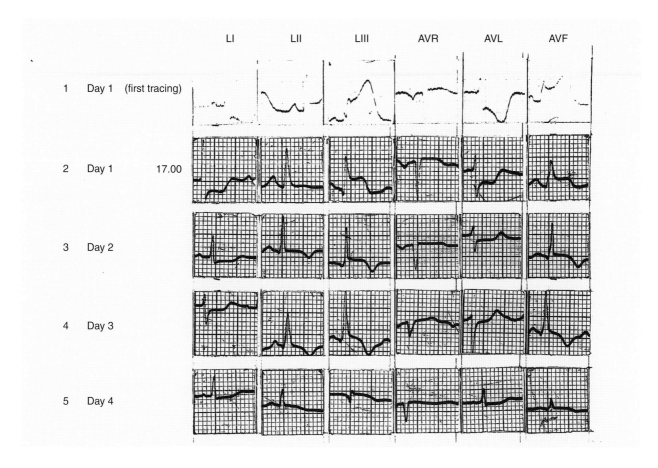

Figure 4.9 *Inferior wall pre-infarct syndrome with ischaemia Grade 3. In panel 2, the first stage of reperfusion is detected in lead LIII. Note the qR pattern in lead LIII, rS in AVL, and Rs in LI. In panel 3, stage 2 of reperfusion is evident in lead LIII. The posterior hemiblock-like patterns persist. In panel 4, the tracing shows an increase in the R wave in LIII and a deepening of the S wave in AVL (signs of re-ischaemia). Panel 5 shows the disappearance of the posterior hemiblock-like pattern. There is a qR pattern in lead LIII and no S wave in AVL or LI.*

without tachycardia. The ECG shows the severe haemodynamic alteration occurring in the left ventricle.[11] This haemodynamic alteration is a sudden and severe increase of the left ventricular end-diastolic pressure. It is caused by a dysfunction of the left ventricle, which in turn is caused by a global reduction in the coronary blood flow. The extremely high diastolic blood pressure severely affects the subendocardial layer.[12]

In circumferential ischaemia, reduction in coronary flow is seen in the whole subendocardium but no significative alteration is seen in the epicardial layer.[12] This dramatic process may develop in less than 30 minutes. The clinical picture starts with orthopnoea and cyanosis and rapidly develops into a picture of severe pulmonary oedema.

CLINICAL AND ECG EVOLUTION OF THE CIRCUMFERENTIAL INFARCTS

The ECG evolution of infarction from circumferential ischaemia is predictable. The first change is a

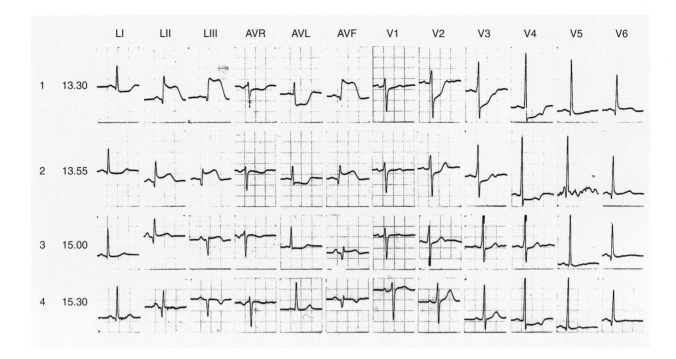

Figure 4.10 *Inferior wall infarction Grade 3. Twenty minutes after thrombolytic therapy (panel 2), the first stage of reperfusion is noted—ST segment elevation of 2 mm and upright T waves of 5 mm in amplitude in inferior leads. In panel 3, 65 minutes later, stage 2 of reperfusion was evident, characterized by 1 mm ST segment elevation and inverted T waves. In panel 4, the ST segment in lead LIII is isoelectric and the T waves are inverted (complete reperfusion). Note the concomitant changes in the ST segment and the T waves in the reciprocal leads (leads AVL, V2, and V3). Note that in this case the ECG signs of complete reperfusion evolved rapidly over only 2 hours.*

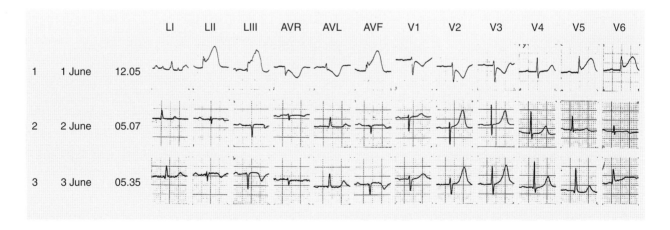

Figure 4.11 *Ischaemia Grade 3 in a patient with posterolateral wall pre-infarct syndrome. In panel 2, approximately 17 hours after the initial ECG, the second stage of reperfusion is evident, characterized by slight ST segment elevation in lead LIII and inverted T waves. The following morning (panel 3), complete reperfusion was evident, characterized by an isoelectric ST segment. In contrast to Fig. 4.10 complete reperfusion evolved over several days.*

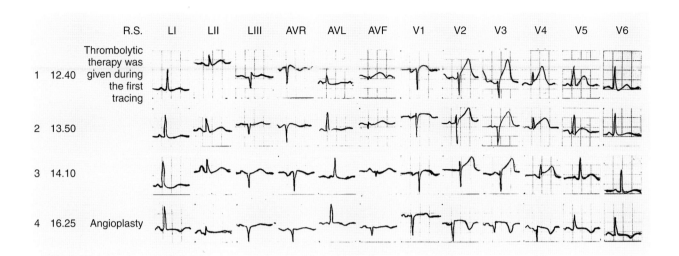

Figure 4.12 *Anterior infarction with ischaemia Grade 2. After thrombolytic therapy there are no signs of reperfusion by ECG. In panel 4, immediately after successful angioplasty in which flow was restored, there are the typical ECG signs of reperfusion with the appearance of the characteristic reperfusion Q waves.*

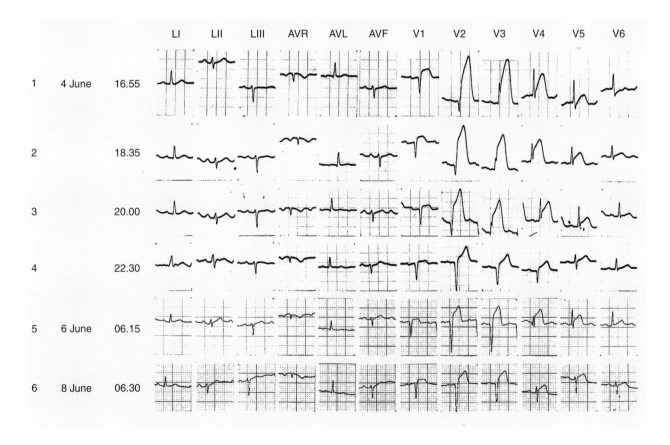

Figure 4.13 *An example of non-reperfusion q waves. Note the progressive deepening of the QS in leads V2 and V3, and the persistent ST segment elevation with upright T waves. The QS in lead V2 in panel 5 is about 18 mm in depth.*

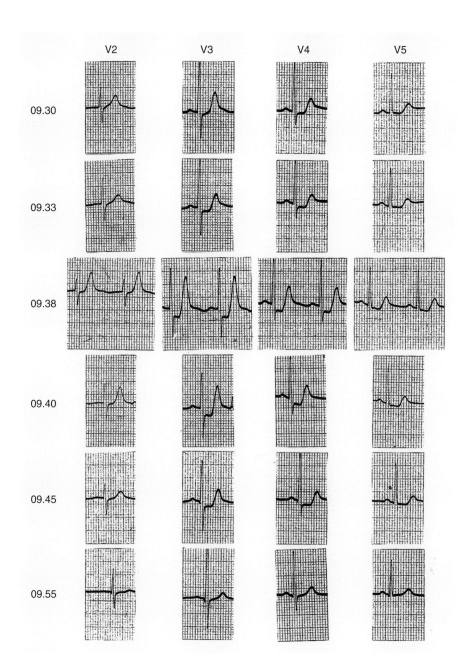

Figure 4.14 *These tracings show the gradual development of tiny q waves in a patient with regional subendocardial ischaemia. Note the ST segment depression with tall and peaked T waves and gradually the appearance in anterior leads of new tiny q waves in leads V2 and V3.*

marked depression of the ST segment with negative T waves maximal in leads V4 and V5. After 10–15 minutes, during which the clinical picture deteriorates, signs of incomplete left bundle branch block (LBBB) with frontal right axis deviation appear. The incomplete LBBB indicates the onset of ventricular dilatation (*Fig. 4.18*), and it progresses toward a complete LBBB. When the left ventricle is dilated, the branches of the left bundle are elongated by traction. The left bundle is fixed in the 'fibrous skeleton'[13] between the rings of the aortic and mitral valves.

Right axis deviation is a very common phenomenon in acute ischaemia and is associated in most

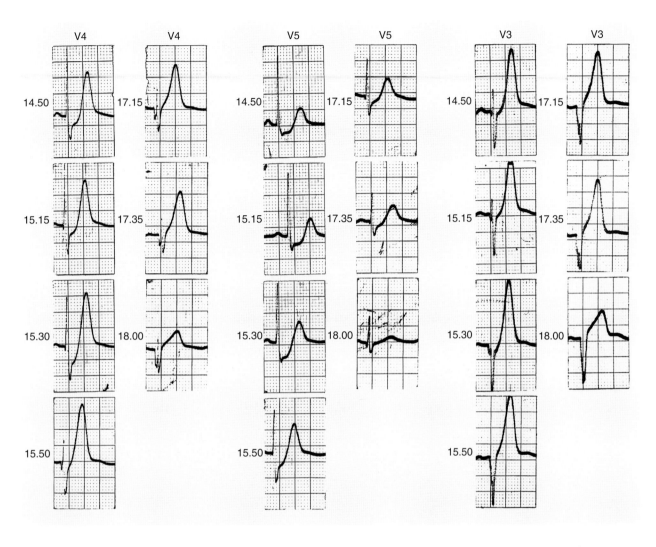

Figure 4.15 *These tracings show the gradual development of an embryonic QrS wave in a patient with regional subendocardial ischaemia in lead V3. Note that in lead V4 the complex that develops is different; there is a QRS complex that develops. In lead V5, there is a decrease in the R waves and the development of a tiny q wave.*

cases with circumferential ischaemia. It appears in a transient and acute form in patients with inferoposterior ischaemia (*Fig. 4.19*).[14]

Clinically, the patient deteriorates rapidly when the diastolic pressure is below 60 mmHg. The ventricular diastolic pressure is very high, above 40 mmHg. When the ventricular and the aortic pressure are balanced, intramyocardial coronary flow ceases. If the LBBB does not disappear the patient often dies suddenly (non-arrhythmogenic sudden death) (*Fig. 4.20*).[15]

Circumferential ischaemias affect most notably the myocardial function in diastole. Treatment by beta-agonists is not recommended because they stimulate systolic contraction and increase the heart rate. They are unnecessary and harmful. Instead, drugs that stimulate the alpha-1-receptors, such as metamerinol (aramine) or noradrenaline, are recommended to increase the aortic diastolic pressure and to restore the diastolic aortoventricular gradient. The first sign of improvement is the disappearance of the LBBB. If the patient survives, the final ECG will show a decrease in the precordial complexes without the appearance of q waves (*Figs 4.21, 4.22*).

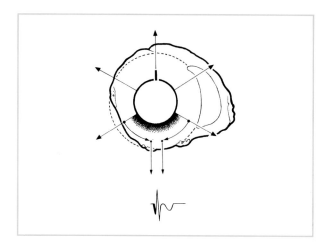

Figure 4.16 *A schematic demonstration of the principles described by Durrer.[10] The tiny q wave is caused by regional subendocardial infarction resulting in retardation of depolarization, permitting the appearance of the opposing vector. The R wave represents the vector progressing toward the lead.*

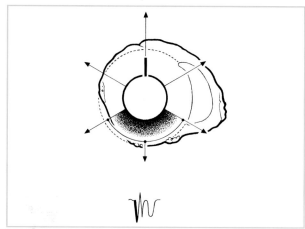

Figure 4.17 *A schematic explanation for the appearance of regional subendocardial ischaemia with deep Q wave and embryonic r waves. The initial vector progresses away from the lead. Subsequently, the epicardial depolarization of the small spared area adjacent to the injured subendocardium results in the appearance of the embryonic r wave.*

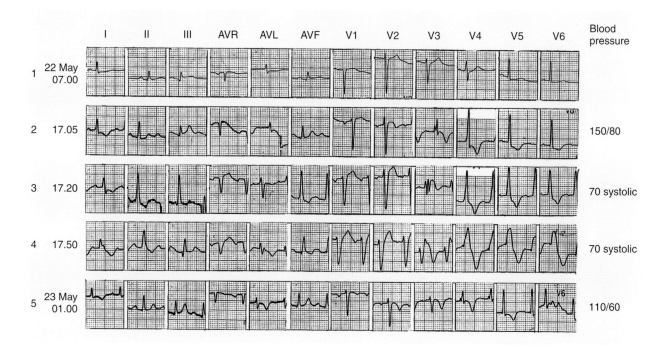

Figure 4.18 *Tracings in circumferential subendocardial infarction. Panel 1, obtained at 07.00, was prior to the ischaemia. Panel 2 was obtained during ischaemia and the appearance of severe shortness of breath. It shows inverted T waves with ST segment depression, with maximal changes in leads V4–V6. Thrombolytic therapy was given at 17.05. Panel 3, 15 minutes later, was recorded as severe pulmonary oedema with hypotension developed. Note the appearance of incomplete left bundle branch block with extreme right axis deviation. There is an increase in size of the R waves in leads LII and LIII and a deep S wave in AVL. In panel 4, complete left bundle branch block developed. In panel 5, obtained 6 hours later when the clinical condition had improved and the haemodynamic parameters were stable, non-Q wave infarction appeared in the precordial leads. Note the changes in the precordial ST–T segments.*

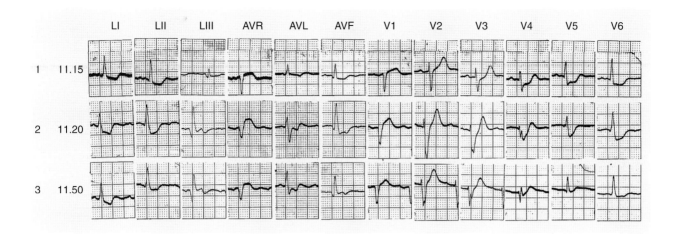

Figure 4.19 *Tracings showing circumferential subendocardial ischaemia with the maximal changes in leads V4 and V5. In panel 2, obtained 5 minutes after the first tracing, the patient deteriorated haemodynamically and the ECG revealed left bundle branch block with right axis deviation. In panel 3, obtained 30 minutes later, these changes persisted and the patient died shortly after.*

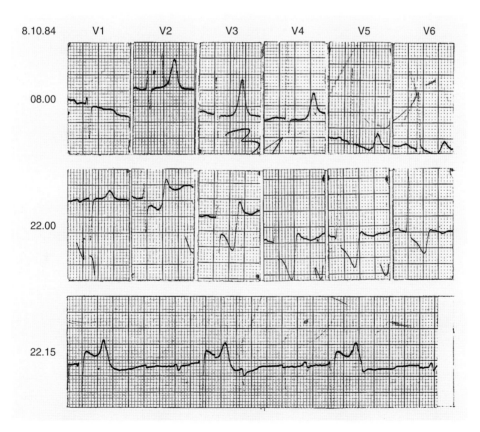

Figure 4.20 *At 08.00, the six precordial leads obtained during routine ECG recordings depict a normal ST segment. At 22.00, after 10 minutes of chest pain, there is severe ST segment depression in leads V4 and V5 with inverted T waves without concomitant tachycardia. Fifteen minutes later the patient was found to have electromechanical dissociation and died (non-arrhythmogenic sudden death).*

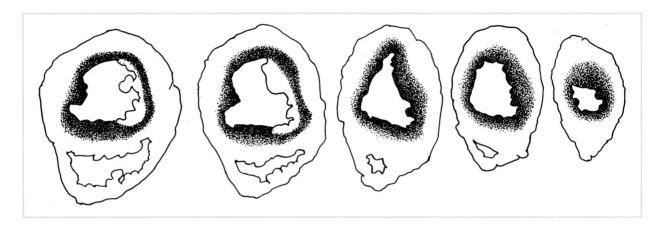

Figure 4.21 *A schematic representation of the myocardium in short-axis in circumferential subendocardial ischaemia. Note the involvement of the subendocardium from the apex to the base. (Adapted from reference 17.)*

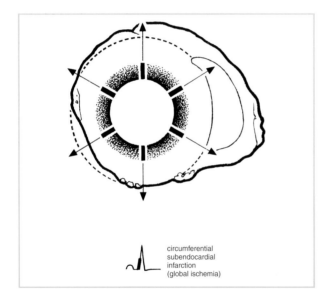

circumferential
subendocardial
infarction
(global ischemia)

Figure 4.22 *A schematic explanation of the absence of the Q wave during circumferential subendocardial ischaemia. In contrast to Fig. 4.9, there are no opposing initial vectors owing to the widespread involvement, and thus there is uniform retardation of the initial vector.*

Pathological anatomy studies of such patients are of great interest. Microscopic study of the heart does not show signs of external haemorrhage, and the surface of the heart is completely normal. A cross-sectional cut shows that the whole subendocardial layer is affected but the external two-thirds of the muscle are normal. This type of infarct was described first by Myers as a 'ring-like subendocardial infarction'[16] and later by Cook as a 'circumferential non-transmural infarction'.[17] The present author has studied six cases of global subendocardial infarction and in each case the same pathological morphology of a total subendocardial lesion was found. Histology shows a severe cellular lesion (cytolysis) in the whole subendocardial layer of the left ventricle, but the external layers show a normal histology (*Fig. 4.23e*). Electron microscopy gives valuable information.

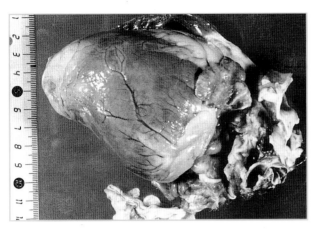

a

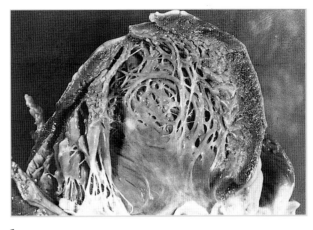

b

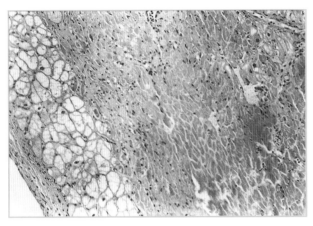

c

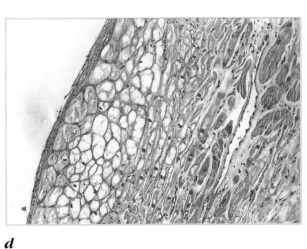

d

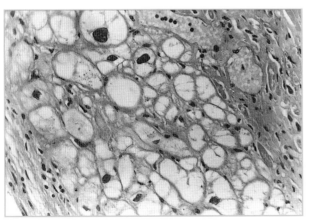

e

Figure 4.23 *A macroscopic specimen from a patient who died from circumferential subendocardial infarction. (a) Note that the epicardial surface seems normal. (b) A vertical cross-section of the left ventricle, however, depicts severe infarction of the subendocardial layer, sparing the epicardial layer. (c and d) High-powered magnification using light microscopy shows that the membrane remains intact but the myocytes in the subendocardial layer are empty, without nuclei. (e) The epicardial layer remains intact. In electron microscopy (×10 000), the few cells with nuclei in the subendocardium appear pyknotic.*

REFERENCES

1. Kondo T, Kubota I, Tachibana H, et al. Glibencamide attenuates peaked T wave in early phase of myocardial ischemia. *Cardiovasc Res* 1996; **31:** 683–7.

2. Burgess MJ, Lux RL. Physiological cisis of the T waves. In: *Advances in Electrocardiography.* (Schlant RC, Hurst JW, eds). New York: Grune and Stratton, 1976.

3. Noma A. ATP regulated K+ channels in cardiac muscle. *Nature* 1983; **305:** 147–8.

4. Chesebro JH, Zoheligi P, Fuster V. Pathogenesis of thrombosis in unstable angina. *Am J Cardiol* 1991; **68:** B2–10.

5. Guyton R, McClenathan JH, Newman GH, et al. Significance of subendocardial ST-segment elevation caused by coronary stenosis in dogs. Epicardial ST-depression, local ischemia and subsequent necrosis. *Am J Cardiol* 1977; **40:** 373–80.

6. Mazzaki U, Miller MJ, Kempess R. Non-uniformity of inner and outer systolic wall thickening in conscious dogs. *Am J Physiol* 1985; **249:** H241–8.

7. Jedeikin LA. Regional distribution of glycogen and phosphorylase in the ventricle of the heart. *Circ Res* 1964; **14:** 202–11.

8. Weiss HR, Sinha AK. Regional O$_2$ saturation of small arteries and vein in canine myocard. *Circ Res* 1978; **42:** 119–26.

9. Dumm RB, Griggs DM. Transmural gradients in ventricular metabolites produced by stopping blood flow in dogs. *Circ Res* 1975; **37:** 438–48.

10. Durrer D, Van Lier AAVV, Buller W. Epicardial and intramural excitation in chronic myocardial infarction. *Am Heart J* 1964; **39:** 765–76.

11. Palacios I, Morvell SB, Powel WJ. Left ventricle end diastolic pressure volume relationship with experimental global ischemia. *Circulation* 1976; **39:** 744–55.

12. Visner M, Aventzen CE, Parresh DG. Effects of global ischemia on the diastolic properties of the left ventricle in conscious dogs. *Circulation* 1985; **71:** 610–19.

13. Lenegre J. Etiology and pathology of bilateral bundle branch block in relation to complete heart block. *Prog Cardiovasc Dis* 1964; **6:** 409.

14. Sclarovsky S, Sagie A, Strasberg B, et al. Transient right axis deviation during acute anterior wall infarction or ischemia: electrocardiographic and angiographic correlation. *Am J Coll Cardiol* 1986; **8:** 27–31.

15. Sclarovsky S, Davidson E, Lewin R, et al. Unstable angina pectoris evolving to acute myocardial infarction. *Am Heart J* 1986; **112:** 459–62.

16. Myers GB, Siars SH, Hivatzka T. Correlation of the electrocardiographic and pathologic finding in ring like subendocardial infarction of left ventricle. *Am J Med Sci* 1951; **222:** 417.

17. Cook RW, Edwards JE, Pruit RD. Electrocardiographic changes in acute subendocardial infarction. *Circulation* 1958; **18:** 603–12.

Chapter 5 The evolving acute myocardial infarction

SUMMARY

In this chapter the different ECG patterns that commonly occur 3 or more days after an acute myocardial infarct are described. In addition, the correlation between these distinct patterns and both invasive and non-invasive examinations is described, and patterns associated with poor outcome are highlighted.

INTRODUCTION

During the first 3 days after an acute myocardial infarct, the ECG may continue to evolve. The ECG changes include those that are expected as well as those that are not.

ECG signs of incomplete reperfusion (qS waves, ST segment elevation, T1 elevation, T2 inversion) or non-reperfusion (qS waves, ST segment elevation, T1 and T2 elevation) may still evolve toward more benign stages. Conversely, the ECGs of patients with a pattern of complete reperfusion may evolve either suddenly or gradually towards more severe patterns, because of a silent and progressive obstruction of the reperfused artery.

During the first few days after myocardial infarction, various pathophysiological processes are initiated, including the release of cytokines, the stimulation of inflammatory cells, and the resorption of necrotic tissue.[1] Collateral circulation may also mature over the first 72 hours.[2] Thereafter, the healing process begins. After about 72 hours, the ECG configuration reaches a stable morphology. Therefore, the ECG recorded on day 3 can be used to predict the changes that will take place during the next 7–10 days. In the following discussion, the author will distinguish between the ECG patterns associated with anterior and inferior infarctions.

THE ECG RECORDED DURING THE THIRD DAY AFTER ANTEROSEPTAL INFARCTION

Three patterns of the evolving anteroseptal infarction can be recognized. They depend on the relationship between the QS waves, the ST segment, and the T waves.

Group A (*Fig. 5.1a*) is characterized by:

- qS waves that are maximally deep in anterior leads V2 and V3;
- isoelectric ST segments in leads V2 and V3; and
- inverted T waves.

Group B (*Fig. 5.1b*) is characterized by:

- qS waves that are maximally deep in anterior leads V2 and V3;
- ST segment elevation of more than 3 mm; and
- positive T1 waves and negative T2 waves.

Group C (*Fig. 5.1c*) is characterized by:

- qS waves that are maximally deep in anterior leads V2 and V3;
- ST segment elevation of more than 5 mm; and
- positive, tall and peaked T1 and T2 waves.

In the following discussion the author will try to describe each pattern further, to correlate the three patterns with the findings in other invasive and non-invasive tests such as echocardiography or angiography, to predict clinical outcome, and to predict the subsequent ECG changes.

GROUP A

The qS waves have special characteristics. The wave is maximally inverted in leads V2 and V3. Generally the depth is 8–12 mm. There is a 'notch wave' in the descending branch of the complex. In leads V4 and

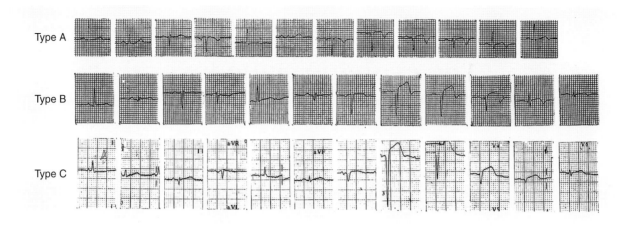

Figure 5.1 *The three distinct types of anterior Q-wave infarction according to the ST–T changes. The top panel shows type A infarction: isoelectric ST segment in the precordial leads and inverted T waves seen maximally in leads V2 and V3 (core of ischaemia), gradually decreasing toward leads V5 and V6. There is a QS wave in lead V2, 8 mm deep, with a notch in the descending limb, which is most evident in lead V3. The amplitude of the standard leads is normal. The middle panel depicts type B infarction: ST segment elevation and T1 over 2 mm in precordial leads, with an inverted T2 wave. The QS wave is 15 mm deep. The bottom panel represents type C: ST segment elevation with upright T waves in all precordial leads. There is a QS wave in lead V2, 25 mm deep. Note the decrease in amplitude in the standard leads. All precordial leads are involved in the process.*

V5, R waves decrease in magnitude or evolve toward a QR pattern; they possibly evolve toward a qS pattern. If the frontal axis is deviated to the left (left anterior hemiblock), RS waves will appear in the left leads V4 and V5. The frontal ventricular complexes do not decrease in size (*Fig. 5.2a*).

The best sign of reperfusion is the ST segment reaching the isoelectric line. If the ST segment is approximately 2 mm in height, this represents incomplete reperfusion (*Fig. 5.3*). T waves are inverted maximally in leads V2 and V3. Inverted T waves may also evolve in leads V4, V5, and V6, but they are less deep.

The echocardiographic findings in group A manifest typical characteristics of type A infarction (see *Fig. 5.2b*):[3]

• the involved area is hypokinetic;
• the involved area maintains its normal thickness or sometimes presents signs of pseudohyper-

trophy caused by the accumulation of fluids in the reperfused area (oedemas);
• there is no expansion in the area affected;
• there are no signs of hyperkinesia of the posterior wall; and
• there is no intracavity thrombus.

In anterior infarction group A, no late potentials are recorded, and therefore the likelihood of complicated ventricular arrhythmias developing is very low (see *Fig. 5.2c*).[4] The patients also usually have normal variability in heart rate (see *Fig. 5.2d*). Over 90% of these patients have a patent infarct-related artery seen on coronary angiography (see *Fig. 5.2e*).[5] The perfusion defect in sestamibi scintigraphy is mild and not extensive (see *Fig. 5.2f*).[6] On multigated angiography (MUGA) the ejection fraction is commonly normal with slight hypokinesia (see *Fig. 5.2b*).

These patients do not have clinical signs of heart

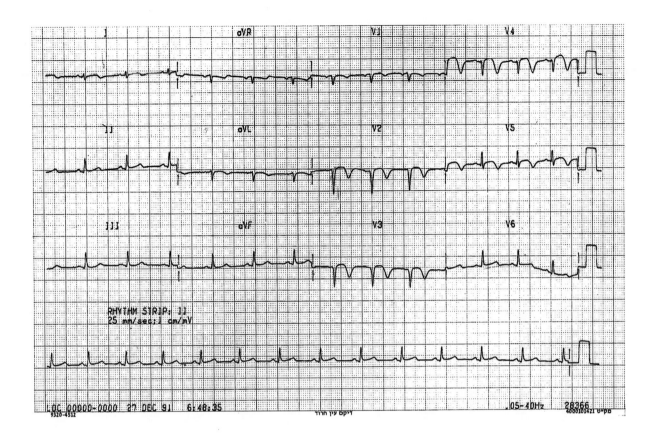

a

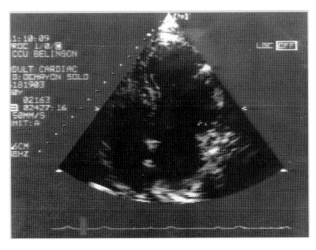

b

Figure 5.2 *(a) Typical type A anterior infarction 3 days after the acute event. (b) Two-dimensional echocardiogram in the four-chamber view showing hypokinesia in the anteroseptal wall and mild hypertrophy of the intraventricular septum. No intraventricular thrombus is evident. (c) Late potential recording. No late potential was seen. (d) Sestamibi scintigraphy demonstrating a small perfusion defect in the anteroapical wall. (e) Multiple-gated acquisition scan of the heart showing mild hypokinesia in the anteroapical wall and a left ventricular ejection fraction of more than 50%. (f) Coronary angiography in the left anterior oblique caudal view showing a severe stenosis in the left anterior descending coronary artery with TIMI 3 flow.*

Continued overleaf

c

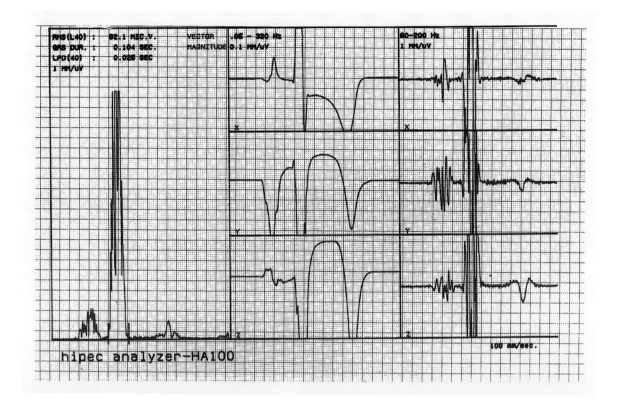

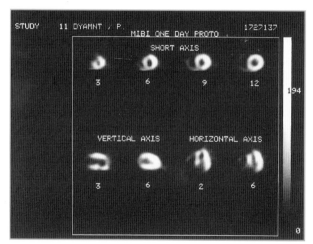

d

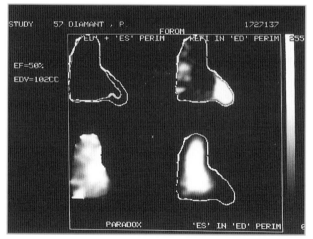

e

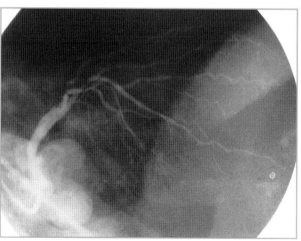

f

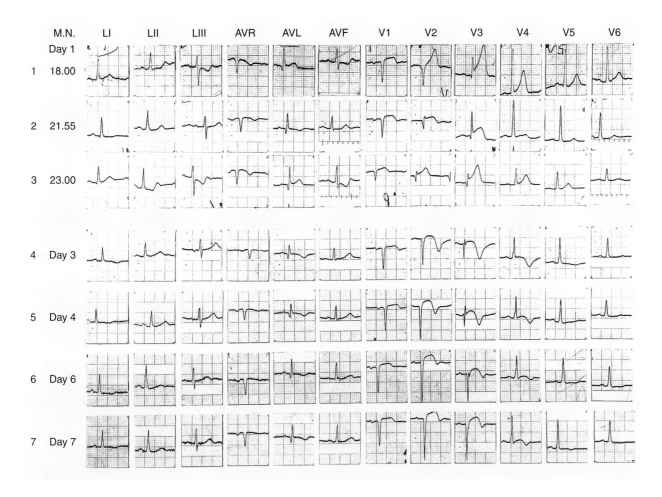

Figure 5.3 *Panels 1 to 3 depict serial ECG tracings of anterior wall pre-infarction with ECG signs indicative of reperfusion stage 1 in panels 2 and 3. Panel 4 demonstrates the typical pattern occurring on Day 3 after type A anterior infarction, but with moderately elevated ST segment elevation. The last three panels demonstrate how the T waves gradually become less inverted. As of Day 7 (bottom panel), there is no more change in the ECG tracings.*

failure (i.e. they have no third heart sound on auscultation), and pericardial friction rubs are rarely heard, but they have a tendency to have painful episodes of re-ischaemia, probably because their coronary lesion is friable and because of the presence of surviving myocardium (*Fig. 5.4*).[7]

The ECG in patients without episodes of re-ischaemia will not change until day 10. The changes that do occur usually signify re-ischaemia. Pseudonormalization of the T waves may be transitory (see *Fig. 5.4*), although occasionally it may persist, indicating re-occlusion of the artery (*Fig. 5.5*).

GROUP B

The QS segment is approximately 15 mm deep, maximally so in leads V2 and V3. In the majority of the cases there is no descending 'notch wave'. R waves in leads V5 and V6 become progressively smaller up to day 3. The ST segment is approximately 4–5 mm in height, in accordance with the upright T1 waves, while T2 waves are inverted. There may be either small inverted T waves (*Fig. 5.6*) or more pronounced inverted T waves (3–4 mm) in leads V2 and V3 (*Fig. 5.7*). It is important to differentiate between these two patterns

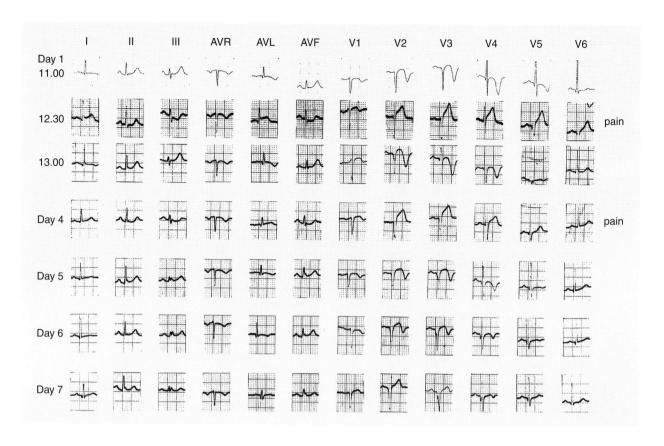

Figure 5.4 *The upper row shows the typical ECG pattern obtained during type A infarction. This pattern was recorded at 11.00. Ninety minutes later, during chest pain, there was re-elevation of the ST segment and the T waves in all precordial leads (second panel), with a return to the baseline tracing 30 minutes later (third panel). During the next day, similar episodes were evident.*

because the former has a course similar to Group A, whereas the latter resembles Group C. T2 waves may be markedly inverted in left precordial leads V4 and V6, whereas in precordial leads V2 and V3 they are slightly negative. Outcome is determined by the pattern in leads V2 and V3, the core of infarction (*Fig. 5.8*).

This group has a distinct evolution of ECG changes. By day 3 or 4, the ST segments and the T waves become taller. By day 9 or 10, the ST segment is elevated, but not to the isoelectric line. The T waves become progressively inverted. These changes

must be distinguished from ischaemia as described for the above group A. These changes are referred to as being 'non-ischaemic second peak', and are probably related to infarct expansion (*Fig. 5.9*).

GROUP C

There are deep QS waves in leads V2 and V3 (18–25 mm). There is no notch in the descending limb. The infarction is extensive and involves several leads. The complexes in the frontal plane are of

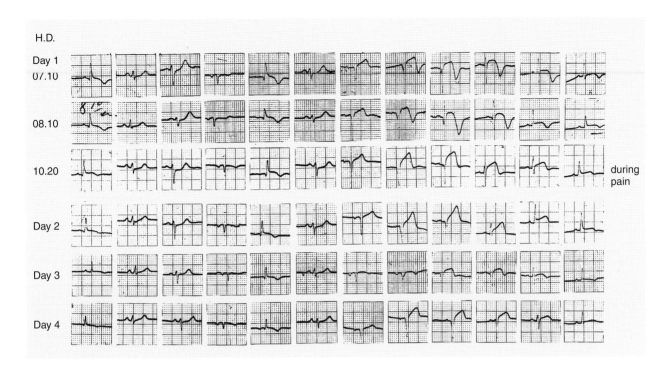

Figure 5.5 *Type A anterior infarction with re-ischaemia evident in the third panel. This re-ischaemia is persistent, in contrast to the recurrent events in Fig. 5.4. This indicates that the artery has reoccluded permanently.*

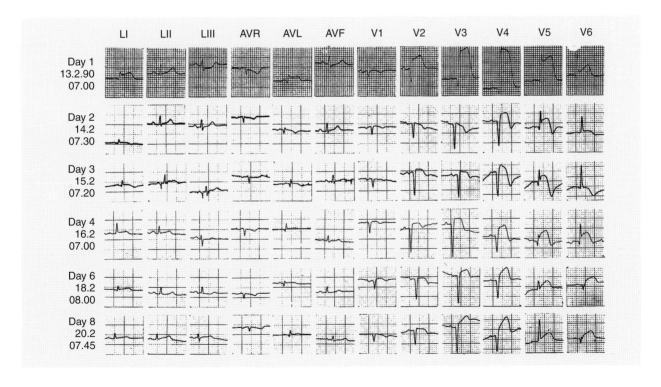

Figure 5.6 *Typical type B infarction. Note that in the second day of the infarction (second panel), there is ST segment elevation in leads V2–V5; and that ST segment elevation develops progressively in the subsequent panels, with the maximal amplitude attained on Day 8 (bottom panel).*

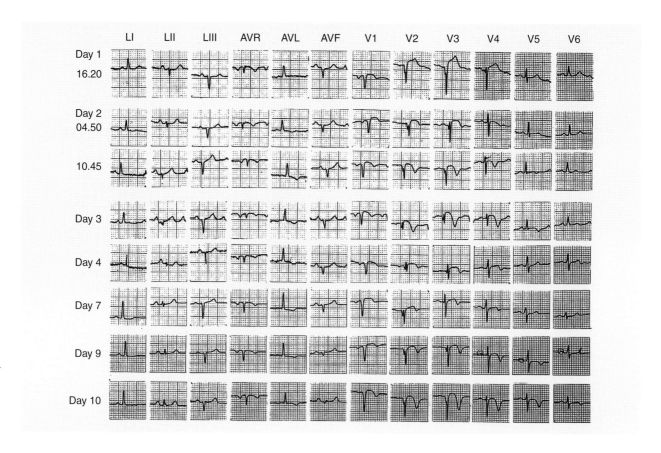

Figure 5.7 *Anterior wall infarction with negative T waves and ST segment elevation of more than 2 mm in the third panel. The evolving ST–T pattern is similar to that seen in group B anterior wall infarction. The pattern of the bottom panel shows a typical infarction with QS wave reperfusion in leads V2 and V3. Note the marked notch in the descending limb of the QS wave, with deep inverted T waves. There is no change in the amplitude of the QRS complex in the frontal plane.*

small size (deep QS in leads V2 and V3 and small standard leads) (*Fig. 5.10a*). The ST–T complex remains greatly elevated (ST segment by 5 mm and the T wave by 10 mm). The leads facing the core of the infarction (leads V2 and V3) are the important leads to follow. The echocardiographic findings (see *Fig. 5.10b*) are:

- septum and apex reduced in their thickness (6–8 mm);
- a marked dyskinetic area;
- dilatation of the affected area;

- hyperkinesia of the opposite area; and
- intracavity thrombus.

Coronary angiography usually reveals an obstructed or suboccluded (TIMI flow 1) artery (see *Fig. 5.10c*).

Patients in group C commonly have positive late potentials (see *Fig. 5.10d*). Hence they are prone to suffer from severe, life-threatening ventricular arrhythmias. Heart rate variability is severely reduced. On sestamibi scintigraphy, there is a severe perfusion impairment, which is often extensive

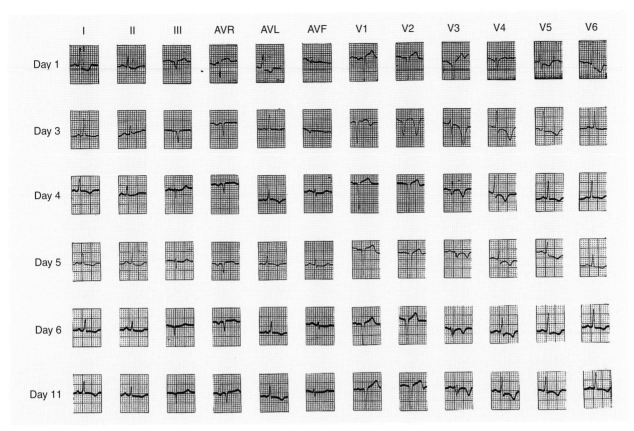

Figure 5.8 *On Day 3 after the acute event, a type A infarction is evident. Note that in leads V3–V6 there is an isoelectric ST segment with an inverted T wave. However, in the core of the infarction (lead V2), there is re-elevation of the ST segment and upright T waves.*

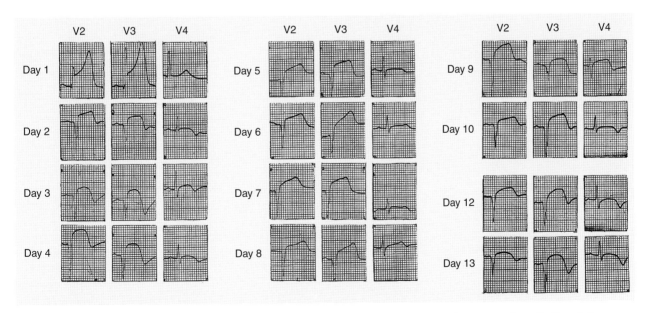

Figure 5.9 *ECG evolution of type B infarction. On Day 1 anterior wall pre-infarct syndrome is evident. By Day 3 there are maximally inverted T waves in leads V2 and V3 and significant ST segment elevation (more than 5 mm). From Day 4 onwards, there is less T wave inversion and less ST segment elevation. From Days 6–8, upright T waves and ST segment elevation are evident, maximally so in leads V2 and V3. From Day 10 onwards, there is progressive inversion of the T wave. On Day 13, there is an inverted T wave with less ST segment elevation.*

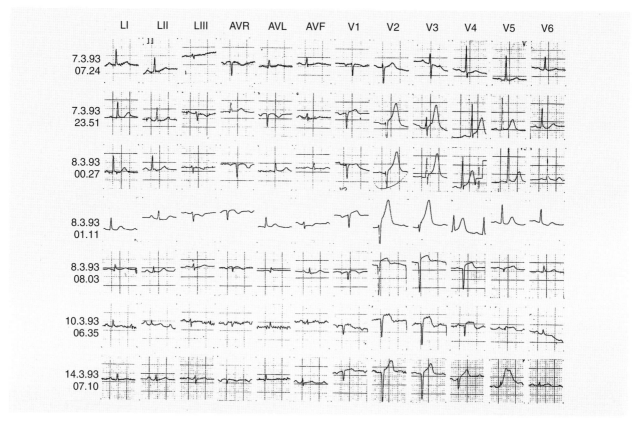

a

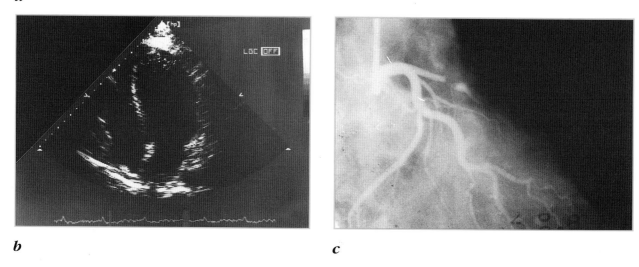

b   *c*

Figure 5.10 *Type C infarction. (a) The typical ECG pattern of type C infarction. There is ST segment elevation with upright T waves throughout the period shown. A QS wave of 20 mm appeared in leads V2 and V3. Note the absence of the notch in the descending limb of the QS wave. Note also the progressive decrease in the amplitude of the frontal leads. (b) The typical two-dimensional echocardiogram in this type of infarction. Severe dyskinesia of the anteroapical wall is evident. The septum is thin. An intracavitary thrombus is detected. (c) Coronary angiography in the right anterior oblique view demonstrating total obstruction of the left anterior descending coronary artery. (d) Late potential recording demonstrating a marked late potential. (e) Sestamibi scintigraphy demonstrating a severe impairment in uptake in the anteroseptal and lateral walls. (f) Multiple-gated acquisition scan of the heart showing severe akinesia with reduced left ventricular ejection fraction.*

d

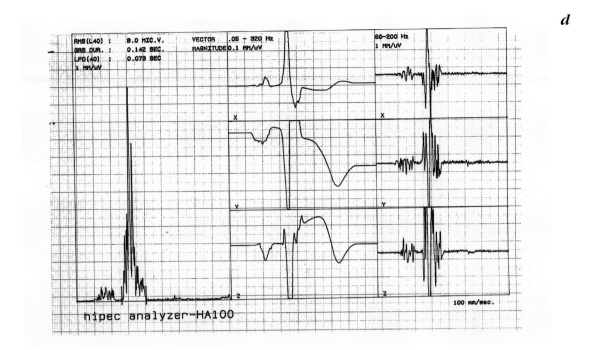

e

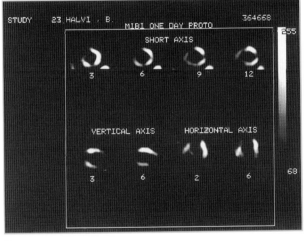

f

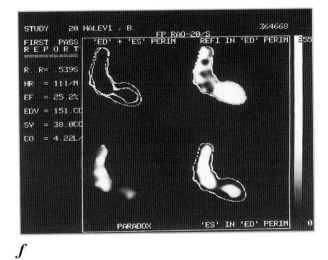

(see *Fig. 5.10e*). Multiple-gated acquisition scanning usually reveals a severely dyskinetic area with a low ejection fraction (see *Fig. 5.10f*).

Clinically, these patients often have heart failure, including the appearance of a third heart sound or a gallop rhythm. Pericardial friction rubs are frequently heard. Re-ischaemia is rare because the myocardium has been so severely damaged, and very frequently the culprit artery is totally obstructed.

The ECG remains stable over time during the first 10 days (*Fig. 5.11*). T waves can become inverted within 10–20 days or up to 6 months after the myocardial infarction, but they do not become inverted in every case (*Figs 5.12, 5.13*).

INFEROPOSTERIOR INFARCTION

The ECG morphology of the QRS complex can be used to evaluate the size of the infarction in infero-posterior infarction. In almost all inferior infarcts a qS wave in lead LIII appears; this lead records the potentials of the inferior wall. The morphology of lead LII appears in inferoposterior infarcts because it records the potentials of the posterolateral wall, which may or may not be seriously involved in the necrotic process. However, it is possible to use the morphology of this lead to evaluate the size of the infarct (*Fig. 5.14*).[8]

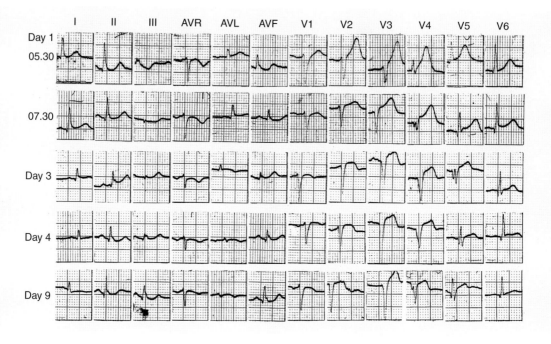

Figure 5.11 *The typical evolution of type C infarction. Deep QS waves more than 20 mm deep are shown in lead V3 from Day 9. Note the ST segment elevation and upright T waves and the progressive decrease of QRS complex in the standard leads.*

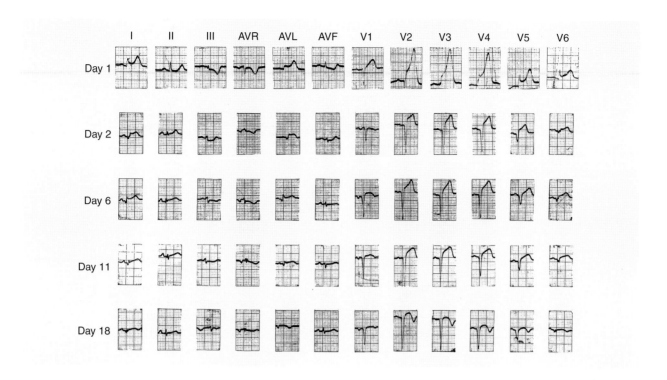

Figure 5.12 *Another example of type C infarction with deep QS waves in leads V2 and V3, and ST segment elevation in the first 18 days. Note the decrease in the amplitude of the QRS complex in the frontal plane.*

Using the ratio Q:R in lead LII, three types of infarction (in the absence of left anterior hemiblock, posterior hemiblock, complete right or left bundle branch block) can be recognized (*Fig. 5.15*):

- Group A, in which q < R;
- Group B, in which q = R; and
- Group C, in which Q < r.

GROUP A

All patients with inferior wall infarction present with QS pattern in lead LIII. In this group, the q waves in lead LII are always smaller than the R waves, indicat-

ing that the posterolateral wall is not involved in the process. R waves in lead LII reveal depolarization of the posterior wall. R waves in leads LI and AVL remain either at the same magnitude or increase from their original size. Potentials in lead AVL are enlarged because potentials of the inferior wall are smaller. In this type of infarction, the precordial leads do not participate in the process because the infarct is localized in the frontal plane. The R waves in leads V5 and V6 are not altered and neither is the size of the S waves in leads V1 and V2.

On echocardiography, there is hypokinesia that is limited to the inferior wall with normal contraction of the lateral and anteroseptal walls (*Fig. 5.16a*). In 60% of these patients, there is involvement of the

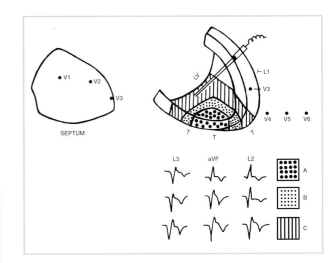

Figure 5.13 *A schematic explanation of the appearance of a notch in the QS wave. In contrast to the normal vectors responsible for the QRS complex (a), the diagram in (b) depicts the vectors that occur with the appearance of the notch: there is a decrease in the very early vectors permitting the appearance of the Q wave, but the surviving myocytes within the infarct are responsible for the opposing vectors which explain the lack of a deep S wave. The diagram in (c) explains the type C infarction. The deep S wave occurs because there are no vectors because of the lack of surviving myocytes. The opposing vector is thus accentuated owing to the disappearance of the 'cancellation phenomenon'. In (d) the vectors indicate a posterior wall infarction, which is manifested by ECG as an increase in the amplitude of the R wave in anterior precordial leads. In (e), the opposing vectors are 'cancelled out', resulting in small amplitude QRS complexes.*

Figure 5.14 *A schematic representation of the different types of inferior infarctions. From type A to type C there is an increase in the extent of the damage.*

right ventricle. Usually there is an obstruction of the posterior descending coronary artery. In 80% of these patients, this artery arises from the right coronary artery; but the right artery has to be of reduced

size and not supplying the posterolateral wall for this type of infarction to occur.

A high percentage of these patients have inverted T waves in lead LIII and isoelectric ST segments in lead LIII only. T waves may become inverted in leads LII and AVF only several days later (*Fig. 5.17*). The mortality in these cases is very low. It is important to seek the ECG changes because they are often confined to only one lead, making the condition difficult to diagnose (*Fig. 5.18*).

GROUP B

The Q waves are equal in size to the R waves. These infarcts are of a greater size than those described above; they involve a portion of the posterior wall. The lateral wall is not involved. Patients suffering from these infarcts are an intermediate group between groups A and C, and they may show ECG, echocardiographic and clinical parameters intermediate between the other two groups. On echocardiography, the hypokinesia is more diffuse and extensive (*Fig. 5.16b, 5.19*).

GROUP C

The Q waves are larger than the R waves. The whole posterior wall is involved and the left lateral wall is

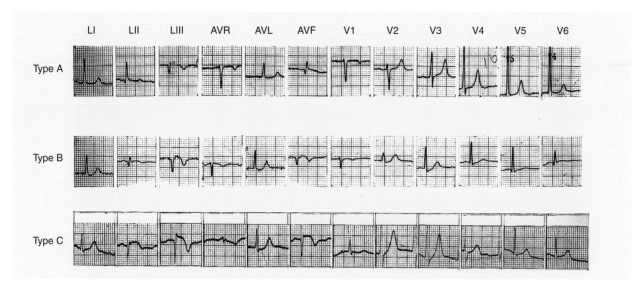

Figure 5.15 *The three types of inferior infarctions according to the morphology in lead LII. In type A infarcts, there is a qR pattern in lead LII. Leads V1, V5 and V6 are not involved. In type B infarcts, the q is equal in size to the R wave in lead LII. Note the positivation of the R wave in lead V2, and the involvement in lead V6. In type C infarcts there is a QR wave in lead LII. Note the significant R wave and the small S wave in lead V1 as well as the involvement in lead V6.*

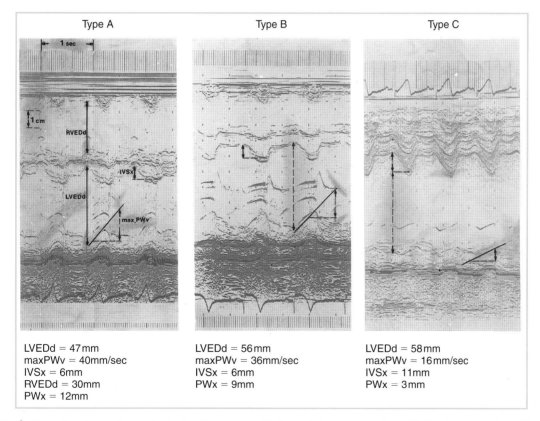

LVEDd = 47 mm
maxPWv = 40 mm/sec
IVSx = 6 mm
RVEDd = 30 mm
PWx = 12 mm

LVEDd = 56 mm
maxPWv = 36 mm/sec
IVSx = 6 mm
PWx = 9 mm

LVEDd = 58 mm
maxPWv = 16 mm/sec
IVSx = 11 mm
PWx = 3 mm

Figure 5.16 *M-mode echocardiography in the three types of inferior infarctions. In type A infarcts, there is hypokinesia of the inferior wall, normal contraction of the septum, and an enlarged right ventricle. Right ventricular infarction is common among type A infarctions, occurring in 60% of this type of infarct. In type B infarcts, there is more extensive hypokinesia in the inferior wall, and the right ventricle is normal in dimensions. In type C infarcts, there is dyskinesia of the posterior wall, left ventricular dilatation, and hyperkinesia of the septum.*

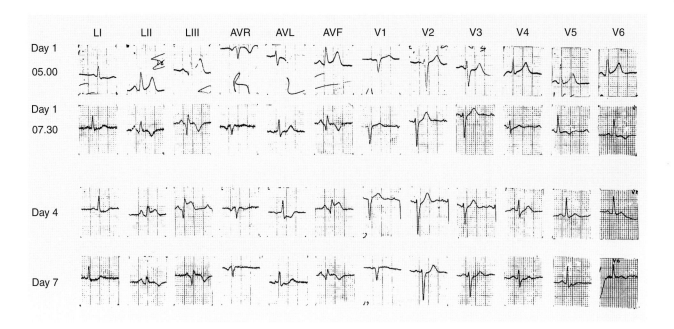

Figure 5.17 *Typical tracings obtained from a patient with type A infarction with signs of complete reperfusion—negative T waves and an isoelectric ST segment. In the third panel, a tracing obtained on Day 4 depicts re-ischaemia, manifested by ST segment elevation in the inferior leads and ST segment depression in lead AVL. The ST segment elevation in lead V1 denotes right ventricular involvement. After the acute ischaemia, type A infarction evolved with a complete reperfusion pattern.*

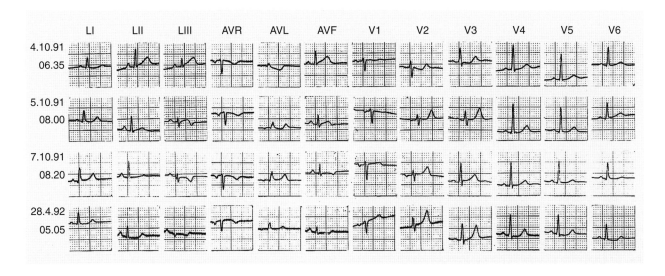

Figure 5.18 *ST segment elevation is seen only in lead LIII in the inferior wall, and a qs pattern is seen only in lead LIII in this variation of type A infarct.*

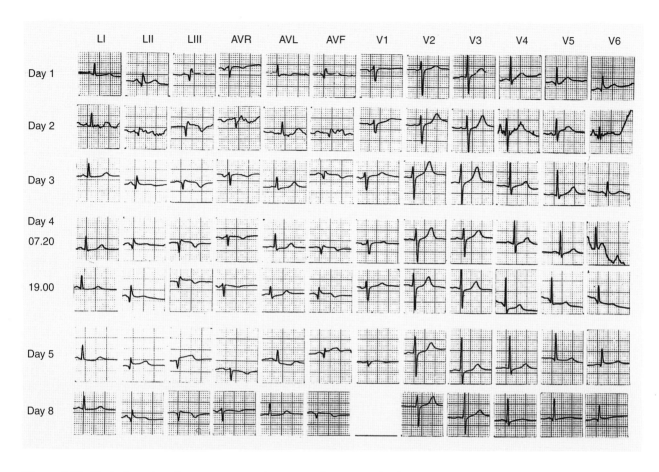

Figure 5.19 *Typical tracings from a patient with type B infarction. In lead LIII, there is a gradual appearance of ST segment elevation and a progressive decrease in the amplitude of the T wave inversion. On Day 5, ST segment elevation with upright T waves was noted (non-ischaemic second peak). By Day 8, the T waves are inverted again in lead LIII with an isoelectric ST segment. Note that the T waves in lead LII are persistently upright.*

also compromised. Because the posterior wall is projected in the anteroposterior plane, the effects of the infarct are also seen in the anterior leads (see *Fig. 5.16c*).

Another ECG parameter seen in this group is the participation of the lateral complexes. These become smaller or develop Q waves because the upper posterior wall is an anatomical continuation of the lateral wall and the two share a common circulation. In leads V1 and V2, S waves become smaller and the ratio R:S is altered in favour of the R waves, indicating the disappearance of the 'cancellation phenomenon' and revealing the anterolateral vectors (see *Fig. 5.13*). Frequently, the frontal complexes become noticeably smaller owing to the expansion of the infarct toward the upper lateral wall (leads LI, AVL, V5, and V6) (*Fig. 5.20*).

The echocardiogram in patients with inferoposterior wall infarction group C shows typical characteristics (see *Fig. 5.16c*):

- extensive dyskinesia or hypokinesia of the inferoposterolateral wall;
- hyperkinesia of the anteroseptal wall;
- a large left ventricular end-diastolic dimension.

These infarcts are generally caused by an occlusion of a circumflex artery or a right dominant artery (especially a predominant artery).

The prognosis for these patients is worse than for patients in groups A and B. They often develop pulmonary oedema, and sudden death is common.

In inferoposterior infarcts the ratio between the ST segment and the T waves has to be considered, with the same subgroups as in the anteroseptal infarcts.

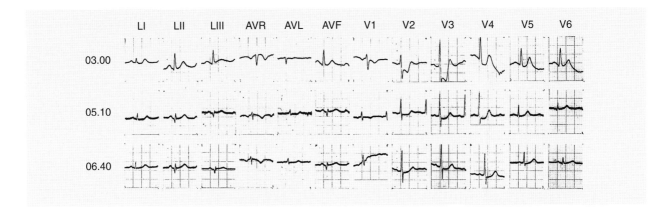

Figure 5.20 *Type C infarction. The upper row demonstrates a tracing in the pre-infarct stage with ECG signs of left circumflex obstruction. In the second row, it is evident that type C infarction has evolved. Note the decreased amplitude in the standard leads, as well as in leads V5 and V6, and the increase in the amplitude of the R waves in leads V1 and V2.*

Thus, in group A inferior infarction, the changes in the ST–T complex frequently correspond to group A anterior infarction (see *Fig. 5.17*) and in group C inferior infarction, the changes in the ST–T complex are similar to those seen in group C anterior infarction.

LEFT ANTERIOR HEMIBLOCK APPEARING DURING THE EVOLVING INFEROPOSTERIOR WALL INFARCTION

Left anterior hemiblock accompanying inferior infarction may be an unrelated finding or a complication of the infarction. Because left anterior hemiblock is a common finding often unrelated to coronary artery disease, it is therefore also common among patients who develop inferior infarction. However, the presence of left anterior hemiblock may make the diagnosis of inferior infarction difficult. If there is antecedent left anterior hemiblock, there are three possible patterns in the ECG:[9]

- the disappearance of R waves in the inferior leads, that is a QS wave; in inferior infarction without antecedent left anterior hemiblock there is always a qr pattern (*Fig. 5.21*);
- a small q wave in lead LII, that is, a qRS complex; by definition, left anterior hemiblock in lead LII must be rS, and therefore the presence of a q wave of any magnitude is always an indication of inferior infarction in a patient with left anterior hemiblock (*Fig. 5.22*); and
- the R waves in lead LII are smaller than the R waves in lead LIII; in left anterior hemiblock without infarction, the R waves in lead LII are taller (*Fig. 5.23*).

The acute development of left anterior hemiblock during infarction is of prognostic significance (see *Fig. 5.8*). In inferior infarction there are two vectors—QR. If three vectors appear in lead LII—QRS—this is a sign of the new appearance of left anterior hemiblock. Left anterior hemiblock complicating inferior infarction is associated with severe disease in the left anterior descending coronary artery system.[10]

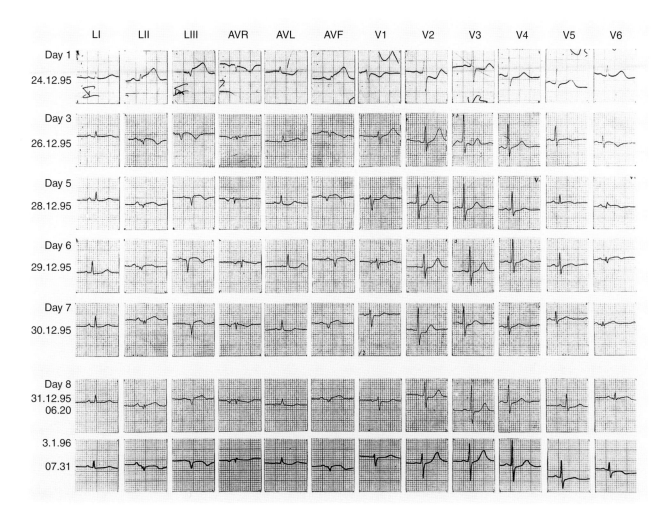

Figure 5.21 *Antecedent left anterior hemiblock in a patient who goes on to develop an inferior wall infarction in the upper row. Note the disappearance of the R waves (QS pattern) in leads LII, LIII, and AVF.*

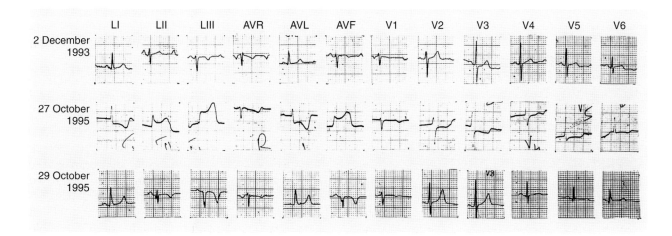

Figure 5.22 *Antecedent left anterior hemiblock in a patient who develops inferior wall infarction. Note that after reperfusion (third panel) there is a qRS pattern in lead LII.*

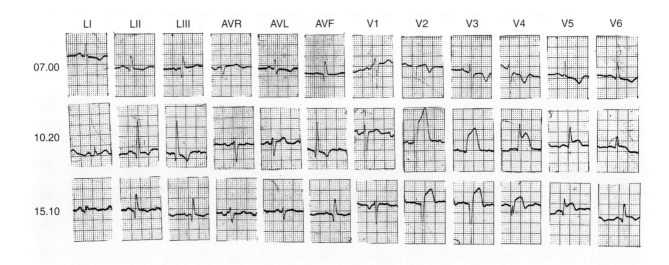

Figure 5.23 *Antecedent left anterior hemiblock in a patient who develops inferior wall infarction in the upper row. There are ECG signs of left circumflex obstruction. Note the disappearance of the R wave in lead LII but not in either LIII or AVF (r in lead 3 is greater in amplitude than r in lead 2). These are signs of a new left posterior hemiblock.*

Figure 5.24 *ECG tracings of a patient with an acute obstruction in the left anterior descending coronary artery supplying collateral circulation to the right posterior descending coronary artery distal to an occluded right coronary artery. Note the inverted T waves in the precordial leads in the top panel. The middle panel depicts anterior wall pre-infarct syndrome. There is right axis deviation with a left posterior hemiblock-like pattern. Note the increase in the R waves in the inferior leads with inverted T waves, and the deepening of the S wave in lead AVL. In the bottom panel, the signs of reperfusion are accompanied by the disappearance of the left posterior hemiblock-like pattern.*

NEW RIGHT AXIS DEVIATION IN ANTERIOR WALL INFARCTION

During acute anterior infarction there are two distinct patterns of right axis deviation in the frontal plane, each with its own pathophysiological explanation. The first pattern entails a posterior hemiblock-like pattern: qR in leads LIII and AVF and RS in AVL with or without an ·S wave in lead LI.[11] This pattern appears commonly during the acute stage of ischaemia or during re-ischaemia. Upon restoration of perfusion, this pattern may disappear, but sometimes it persists. The pathophysiology of this pattern is that the left anterior descending coronary artery is acutely occluded. This artery subtends the area supplied by the posterior descending coronary artery (*Fig. 5.24*).

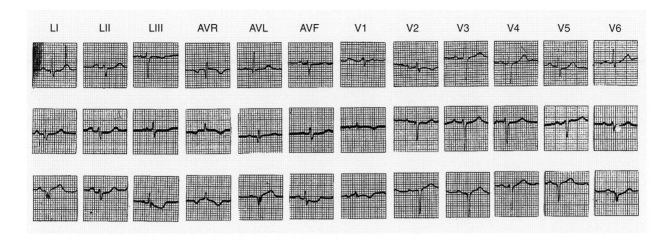

Figure 5.25 *Baseline ECG (top panel) shows extreme left axis deviation reflecting left anterior hemiblock. The middle panel shows a tracing after an acute lateral infarction. Note the appearance of deep Q waves and a decrease in the R waves in leads LI, AVL and the precordial leads. Note the increase in the R waves in lead LIII and AVF. There is no change in the pattern in lead LII. The bottom panel shows a rightward shift in the axis during extensive anterolateral wall infarction. Despite the presence of left anterior hemiblock, there is a shift to the right, owing to the involvement of the high anterolateral wall.*

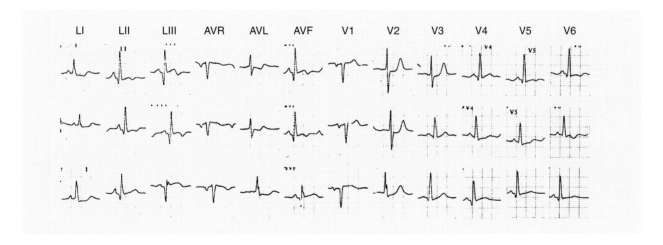

Figure 5.26 *ECGs of an inferior wall infarction in the reperfusion stage. There is a qR pattern in leads LII and AVF with an RS pattern in lead AVL (posterior hemiblock-like pattern). In the middle panel there are inverted T waves. In the bottom panel, the posterior hemiblock-like pattern disappears, there is a tiny R wave in leads LIII and AVF, and the S waves almost disappear in lead AVL. The T waves in the inferior leads gradually become upright.*

The second pattern occurs in infarctions involving the anterosuperior part of the heart. A QS complex occurs in leads LI and AVL, as well as an increase in the amplitude of the R wave in lead LIII. In contrast to the first pattern, this pattern does not have a qR wave in the inferior leads or an RS wave in lead AVL. The pathophysiology for this pattern is the weakening of the vectors in the anterosuperior areas, enabling the appearance of inferior vectors (*Fig. 5.25*).[12]

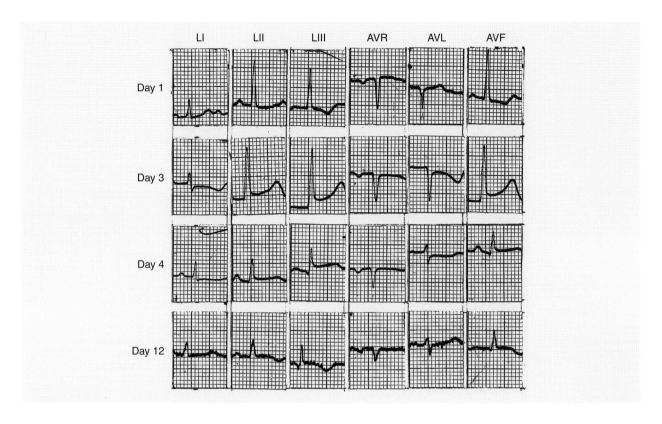

Figure 5.27 *ECGs of an inferior wall infarction with qR waves in leads LIII and AVF, and RS waves in lead AVL. Note the inverted T waves in leads LIII and AVF. Re-ischaemia on Day 3 is shown by additional right axis shift with ST segment elevation and upright T waves in the inferior leads. There are reciprocal changes in leads LI and AVL. The third and fourth panels depict persistent right axis deviation up to Day 12 despite signs of reperfusion.*

NEW RIGHT AXIS DEVIATION IN INFERIOR WALL INFARCTION

As is the case in anterior wall infarction, right axis deviation occurring during inferior infarction has two different patterns. The first pattern, described in Chapter 4, persists during reperfusion and entails a qR wave in the inferior leads and an RS wave in lead AVL. This may persist for a few days or permanently[13] (*Figs 5.26, 5.27*). It is important to stress that during right axis deviation in this pattern, there is a rapid appearance of inverted T waves in lead LIII. When the right axis deviation is resolved, the T waves become upright once again (see *Fig. 5.26*). This is not a sign of pseudonormalization, rather it is related to the axis changes.

The second pattern includes the acute right axis deviation accompanying chest pain. This may occur with or without ST–T changes. This pattern is common during re-obstruction of the right coronary artery (*Fig. 5.28*). Once the ischaemia resolves, the axis deviation is resolved. A persistent deviation denotes a persistent obstruction usually.

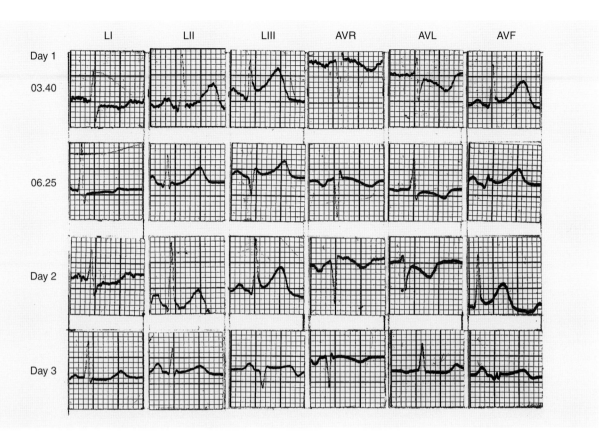

Figure 5.28 *The ECG in the top panel shows acute right axis deviation with a posterior hemiblock pattern. In the second panel, the posterior hemiblock pattern has disappeared. Reperfusion in this case can be seen only by the disappearance of the QRS pattern. The third panel shows re-ischaemia manifested by the reappearance of the posterior hemiblock-like pattern, without significant ST–T changes. The fourth panel demonstrates complete reperfusion with inverted T waves and an isoelectric ST segment in leads LIII and AVF. There are no signs of a posterior hemiblock-like pattern. Note the disappearance of the S waves in lead AVL and the tall R waves in lead LIII.*

REFERENCES

1. Fishbein MC, Maclian D, Ana Maroko P. The histopathological evolution of myocardial infarction. *Chest* 1978; **73:** 843.
2. Schwartz H, Leiboff RH, Brein GB, et al. Temporal evolution of the human coronary collateral circulation after myocardial infarction. *Am J Coll Cardiol* 1984; **4:** 1088.
3. Sagie A, Strasberg B, Imbar S, et al. Value of the electrocardiogram for the prediction of left ventricular mural thrombus in anterior wall acute myocardial infarction. *Am J Cardiol* 1991; **68:** 957–9.
4. Kusniec J, Solodky A, Strasberg B, et al. Relationship between late potentials and the predischarge electrocardiographic pattern in patients with acute myocardial infarction. *Clin Cardiol* 1996; **19:** 645–9.
5. Kusniec J, Solodky A, Strasberg B, et al. The relationship between the electrocardiographic pattern with TIMI flow class and ejection fraction in patients with a first acute anterior wall myocardial infarction. *Eur Heart J* 1997; **18:** 420–5.
6. Adler Y, Zafrir N, Sclarovsky S, et al. Estimation of final infarct size and severity of left ventricular dysfunction by the predischarge electrocardiographic pattern in patients with first acute anterior wall myocardial infarction. Israel Heart Society Meeting, Jerusalem, April 1998.
7. Benjaminov-Sclarovsky F, Sclarovsky S, Birnbaum Y. The predictive value of the electrocardiographic pattern of acute Q wave myocardial infarction and recurrent ischaemia. *Clin Cardiol* 1995; **18:** 710–15.
8. Arditti A, Sclarovsky S, Lewin R, et al. A simplified QRS scoring system for the estimation of the severity of acute inferior wall infarction. *Chest* 1985; **87:** 778–84.
9. Castellanos A, Myerburg RJ. The hemiblocks in myocardial infarction. In: *Criteria of Diagnosis of LAD, LPH in the Presence of Myocardial Infarction.* Century Crofts, New York: Appleton: 1976: Chapter 2.
10. Assali S, Sclarovsky S, Herz I, et al. Importance of left anterior hemiblock development in inferior wall acute myocardial infarction. *Am J Cardiol* 1997; **79:** 672–4.
11. Sclarovsky S, Sagie A, Strasberg B, et al. Transient right axis deviation during acute anterior wall infarction or ischaemia: electrocardiographic and angiographic correlation. *Am J Coll Cardiol* 1986; **8:** 27–31.
12. Sagie A, Sclarovsky S, Strasberg B, et al. Significance of rightward axis shift in acute myocardial infarction. *Am J Noninvas Cardiol* 1991; **5:** 229–34.
13. Lewin L, Sclarovsky S, Strasberg B, et al. Right axis deviation in acute myocardial infarction: clinical significance, hospital evolution and long-term follow up. *Chest* 1984; **85:** 489–93.

Chapter 6   Ventricular arrhythmias in acute ischaemic syndrome

SUMMARY

Ventricular arrhythmias are frequent complications of ischaemic episodes. This chapter describes the different ventricular arrhythmias that may arise during different types of ischaemias, elaborates on the possible pathophysiological mechanisms, and describes the clinical outcomes. In particular, the chapter stresses the importance of the timing of these arrhythmias and the correlation between the stage of ischaemia and the type of arrhythmia that may arise.

INTRODUCTION

The type of arrhythmias that occur in the acute ischaemic syndrome depends on the functional and metabolic changes in the involved area. Therefore there is a relationship between the type of ventricular arrhythmia and the type of acute coronary syndrome. Ventricular arrhythmias that occur in the acute ischaemic process develop because of the dispersion of depolarization in the infarct area between the subendocardium and the epicardium, as well as in the affected and healthy muscle.[1]

As has been explained in earlier chapters, the ECG can recognize the different ischaemic syndromes that are produced by an acute obstruction of an epicardial artery. These ischaemic syndromes are:

- acute transient ischaemia;
- pre-infarct ischaemia;
- non-Q-wave infarction;
- reperfusion Q-wave infarction;
- non-reperfusion Q-wave infarction.

Moreover, the ECG can define the different ischaemic syndromes according to their pathophysiology and anatomic pathology. The ischaemias are:

- regional transmural ischaemias;
- regional subendocardial ischaemias;
- circumferential subendocardial ischaemias.

Each of these ischaemic scenarios may evolve to typical infarcts with different clinical, ECG, and prognostic characteristics.

Subendocardial ischaemias, whether regional or circumferential, do not usually produce fatal arrhythmias. Sudden death as a consequence of circumferential subendocardial ischaemia is caused by acute and severe ventricular dysfunction but not arrhythmias (i.e. non-arrhythmogenic sudden death).[1]

Of the major ventricular arrhythmias that occur in regional transmural ischaemia, most occur during the initial stage of a complete and abrupt obstruction of an epicardial artery or during the sudden relief of the obstruction (reperfusion).[2]

The major arrhythmias that occur during ischaemia are:

- ventricular fibrillation;
- polymorphous ventricular tachycardia;
- ventricular rhythm of intermediate rate—either accelerated idioventricular rhythm or slow ventricular tachycardia.

VENTRICULAR ARRHYTHMIAS DURING PRE-INFARCTION SYNDROME

The ECG can reveal the grade of ischaemia in the regional transmural process and the intensity of the process in the affected area. As has been stressed in earlier chapters, ischaemia Grade 1 and Grade 2 indicate some myocardial protection, either by collateral circulation or by preconditioning, whereas in ischaemia Grade 3 the heart is completely unprotected. Accordingly, regional transmural ischaemia Grade 3 is the main cause of major ventricular arrhythmias, both at the stage of arterial obstruction and during reperfusion.[2]

The most severe ventricular arrhythmia that occurs in the pre-infarct ischaemic syndrome is ventricular

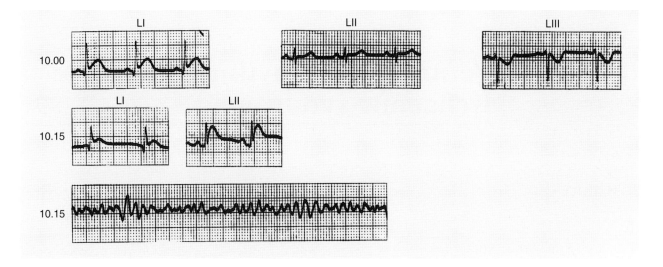

Figure 6.1 *ECG tracings from a patient with acute anterior wall pre-infarct syndrome. The top panel was obtained 10 minutes after the onset of chest pain. ST segment elevation is evident with upright T waves. In lead LIII reciprocal changes are evident. There is minute ST segment elevation in lead LII. The middle panels, obtained 15 minutes later when the pain had worsened, demonstrate increased ST segment elevation in leads LI and LII. The patient immediately developed ventricular fibrillation (bottom panel). Note the rapid, unrecognizable QRS complexes during this fatal arrhythmia.*

fibrillation (*Fig. 6.1*). Ventricular fibrillation may appear in any of the ECG morphologies of the pre-infarct syndrome, but it appears most frequently in ischaemia Grade 3. Ventricular fibrillation appears at the very initial stages of the acute ischaemic process, and there is evidence that it is the main cause of death outside the hospital (see *Fig. 6.1*).[3] It is also often seen in the Emergency Room when the initial stages of the pre-infarct ischaemic syndrome are developing. The ECG characteristics of the arrhythmias that are seen during the continuous recording are:

- an abrupt elevation of the ST segment, and peaked T waves;
- commencement with an extrasystole proximal to the T waves or on top of the T waves, or with rapid bouts of extrasystoles (*Fig. 6.2*);
- small and rapid fibrillation waves with unrecognizable QRS complexes;
- lack of spontaneous reversal but reversal with cardioversion;
- the ECG recorded after cardioversion continues to show signs of acute ischaemia (ST segment elevation and positive T waves) (*Fig. 6.3*);
- repetitive episodes are common, though lidocaine prevents these episodes.

VENTRICULAR ARRHYTHMIAS DURING REPERFUSION

Most ventricular arrhythmias recorded in coronary care units occur during the stage of reperfusion. Reperfusion is the major factor producing the following ventricular arrhythmias:

- ventricular extrasystole;
- polymorphous ventricular tachycardia;
- ventricular arrhythmias of intermediate rate (accelerated ventricular tachycardia and slow ventricular tachycardia).

VENTRICULAR EXTRASYSTOLES DURING PRE-INFARCT ISCHAEMIAS

Different electrocardiographic parameters used to be considered in the evaluation of the risk of extrasystoles in acute ischaemia. These parameters were:

- short, large, fixed or variable coupling;
- high frequency ($\geqslant 5$ per hour)
- appearance of runs.

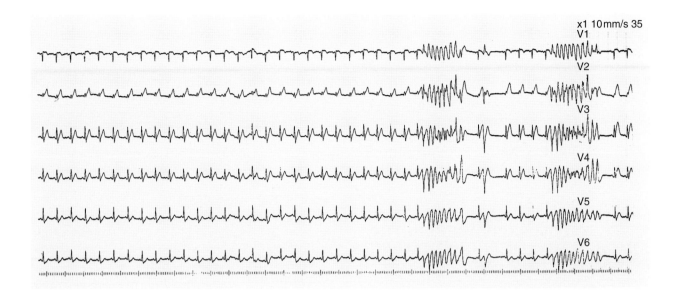

Figure 6.2 *Continuous six-channel ECG tracings at 10 mm/second. Note the maximal ischaemic change in leads V2 and V3. In the third panel, the bout of rapid ventricular dysrhythmia was preceded by an R-on-T phenomenon. Later the same phenomenon occurred without an ensuing dysrhythmia. Note that the first extrasystoles are with an RBBB-like pattern in lead V1, but with a QS pattern in leads V2–V6. Note that after the extrasystoles, the ST segment elevation increased in amplitude. Following this rise in ST segment elevation, an additional extrasystole did cause a ventricular dysrhythmia again with a further subsequent increase in ST segment elevation.*

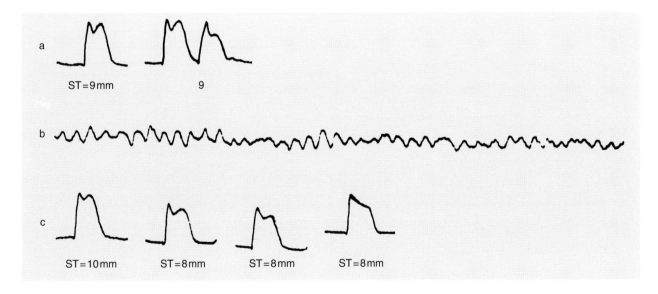

Figure 6.3 *(a) The upper panel demonstrates pre-infarct syndrome with ischaemia Grade 3. The second complex shows extrasystoles developing, although the amplitude of the ST segment elevation is unchanged. (b) Immediately after the ventricular extrasystole, characteristic ventricular fibrillation developed. (c) After cardioversion, there was no significant change in the ST segment, indicating that reperfusion had not been achieved.*

However, in the light of advances of coronary physiology and the possibility of recording simultaneous and continuous 3–6 channel ECG during the acute infarct, two more elements of clinical importance can be introduced:

- the stage of the evolving acute ischaemic process in which the extrasystole appears;
- the morphology of the extrasystole and its relation to the location of the acute ischaemic process.[4]

EXTRASYSTOLES APPEARING IN THE INITIAL STAGES OF THE PRE-INFARCT ISCHAEMIC SYNDROME

In the very early stages of the transmural regional ischaemic process, there is a dispersion of QT in the different layers of the ischaemic zone: the dispersion occurs principally between the endocardium and the epicardium. The ischaemic epicardium becomes hyperpolarized, producing a shortening of phase 2–3 of the action potential in the ischaemic area, while the amplitude of QT in the subendocardial area is not altered.[5] The purpose of this phenomenon is to protect the external layers of the myocardium, but this becomes a 'double-edged sword'—on the one hand it protects the ischaemic myocardium, but on the other hand it induces arrhythmias.[2]

Characteristics of the extrasystoles that appear at the initial stages of the acute ischaemic process include the following:

- they appear at the very early stages of the process;
- they last a short time;
- coupling is short and fixed;
- they are monomorphic, and the location of the process determines the morphology of the extrasystole;
- when they appear as runs, they are of a very high rate (see *Fig. 6.2*);
- they may induce ventricular fibrillation;
- they commonly respond favorably to lidocaine.

These extrasystoles are generally not recorded in the coronary care unit because pre-infarct ischaemias appear more than 1 hour after the onset of the ischaemic process.

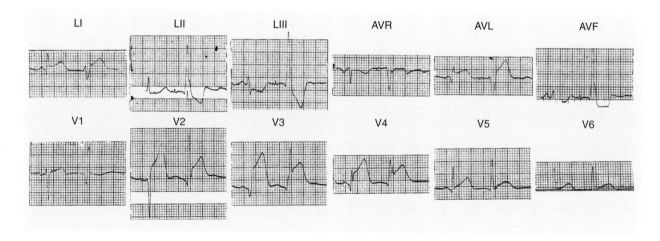

Figure 6.4 *Anterior wall pre-infarction syndrome. The standard leads demonstrate ischaemia in the high anterior wall (ST segment elevation with upright T waves in leads LI and AVL, and ST segment depression with inverted T waves in lead LIII). The extrasystole has severe right axis deviation (rS in AVL and qR in inferior leads). This pattern indicates that the origin of the extrasystole is from the anterior wall. In the leads V1–V6, the first beat shows anterior wall pre-infarction syndrome. The second beat is an extrasystole with an RBBB-like pattern in lead V1. Note that all the extrasystoles in the precordial leads have a prominent R wave, suggesting that the origin is in the upper part of the anterior wall.*

x1 25 mm/s x1 25 mm/s 35 Hz 60 bpm

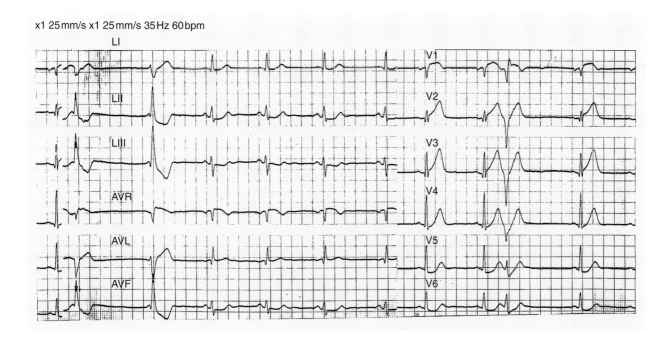

Figure 6.5 *Anterior wall pre-infarction syndrome. In the standard leads, the first two beats are extrasystoles with extreme right axis deviation, suggesting that their origin is from the anterior wall. In the second column, the precordial leads demonstrate a predominant anteroapical pre-infarction. The third beat is an RBBB-like but in leads V2–V4 there is a negative QS pattern, indicating that their origin is from the apex. Note the difference from Fig. 6.4.*

CORRELATION BETWEEN THE MORPHOLOGY OF THE EXTRASYSTOLES AND THE LOCATION OF THE ISCHAEMIC SYNDROME

Anterior wall ischaemias induce extrasystoles with the following pattern:

- right axis deviation; tall R waves in leads LIII, LII and aVF; qS in leads LI and aVL (*Figs 6.4 and 6.5*);
- right bundle branch block (RBBB) in lead V1 with QS (see Fig. 6.2) or R in leads V2–V6 (see *Fig. 6.4*).

In addition, extrasystoles with a left bundle branch block (LBBB) pattern is sometimes seen if the ischaemia is more intense in the right part of the septum, though this is unusual at this stage.

Ventricular extrasystoles appearing in inferior ischaemias show the following morphology (*Fig. 6.6*):

- left axis deviation; qS in leads LII, LIII and aVF;

- R waves in leads LI and aVL;
- qS or qR waves in lead aVR.

The majority of the inferior infarcts have a right or left ventricle involvement; hence they appear with LBBB or RBBB pattern and left axis deviation (see *Fig. 6.6*) unless they arise in the anterior wall of the right ventricle, in which case they show LBBB with right axis deviation (*Fig. 6.7*). If the extrasystoles arise from the apex of the posterior wall, they show an RBBB pattern, but with qS complexes in the rest of the precordial leads.

REPERFUSION ARRHYTHMIAS

After the initial stage of the pre-infarct syndrome, the ischaemic area recovers electrophysiological stability and may remain without any evidence of arrhythmia for a long time (between 30 minutes and up to 4 hours usually). Reappearance of extrasystoles may be the earliest sign of reperfusion. This reappearance

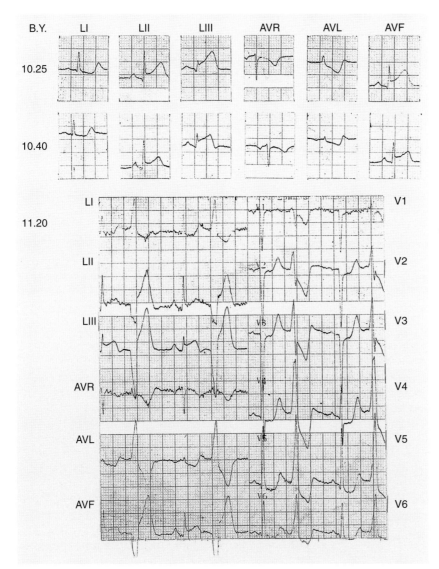

Figure 6.6 *The top panel demonstrates inferior wall pre-infarction syndrome. The second panel depicts a tracing obtained 15 minutes later than the first tracing, showing ECG signs of reperfusion. Subsequent tracings obtained 40 minutes after demonstrate extrasystoles. In the standard leads, the extrasystoles (second and fourth beats) have extreme left axis deviation (R in leads L1 and AVL and QS in the inferior leads), suggesting an origin from the posterior wall. In the precordial leads, the second beat is an extrasystole with an LBBB-like pattern, suggesting that the origin is from the right ventricle. In this case, the right posterior septal area is involved in the ischaemic process.*

may be due to a non-uniformity of the QT waves in the different layers of the ischaemic area. The characteristics of these extrasystoles are very similar to those seen in the pre-infarction syndrome. Frequently the ST segment decreases in amplitude, and the characteristic changes of reperfusion become evident (see *Fig. 6.7*).

POLYMORPHOUS VENTRICULAR TACHYCARDIA

The most dramatic arrhythmias that occur during the phase of reperfusion are the polymorphous ventricular tachycardias,[6] which have very well-defined characteristics:

- they almost always appear with ischaemia Grade 3;
- the ST segment and the T waves decrease toward the isoelectric line immediately after the disappearance of the arrhythmia (*Fig. 6.8*).

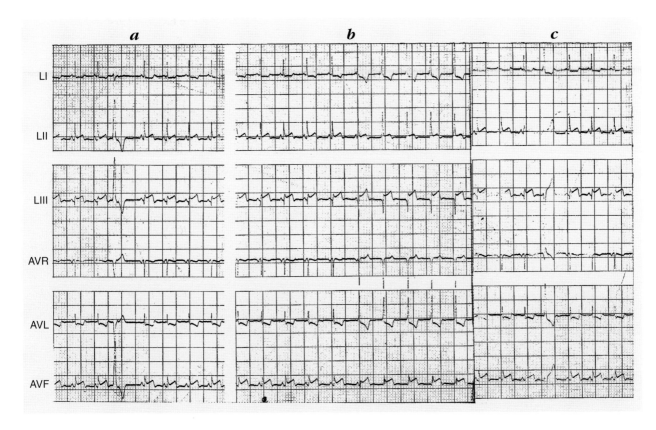

Figure 6.7 *Inferior wall pre-infarction with right ventricular involvement (not shown). (a) The first tracing demonstrates simultaneous six-channel recording. The third beat is an extrasystole with extreme right axis deviation (rS in leads L1 and AVL and qR in the inferior leads). Lead AVR has a QS pattern, suggesting that the origin is the right ventricle. (b) The second tracing, obtained from the same patient, demonstrates a run of six extrasystoles. Note that there was no axis deviation (axis is +40°). In lead AVR, the second to the fifth beats have an LBBB-like pattern. This suggests that the origin of the extrasystoles is from the right ventricle and the lateral walls. Because opposing parts of the heart are stimulated concomitantly, there is no axis deviation. (c) The third tracing shows the third focus of premature ventricular complexes (PVCs) with morphology of left axis deviation (R wave in leads L1 and AVL, rS in leads L2, L3 and AVF). Note the AVR with RBBB-PVCs pattern. This pattern suggests that the origin of the PVCs is from the left ventricle and inferior wall.*

Characteristics of the morphology of the arrhythmia are:

- ventricular complexes of polymorphic type with variable but well-recognized QRS complexes;
- a ventricular rate of about 150–300 beats per minute;
- *torsade de pointes* (intermittent positive and negative complexes appearing) (*Figs 6.9* and *6.10*);
- repetitive polymorphic episodes that sometimes have the same serial morphology during recurrent episodes, i.e. the serial beats during one episode may resemble those in another episode;

- persistence, disappearing only with cardioversion, although they sometimes stop spontaneously (*Fig. 6.11*);
- lidocaine does not prevent them;
- there are no additional episodes following the ECG signs of reperfusion;
- reoccurrence is possible during new episodes of re-ischaemia and reperfusion.

These arrhythmias must be differentiated from the polymorphous ventricular tachycardias that appear in the late stages (after 7 days) of the extensive anterior infarcts—these are malignant processes that usually end with death.

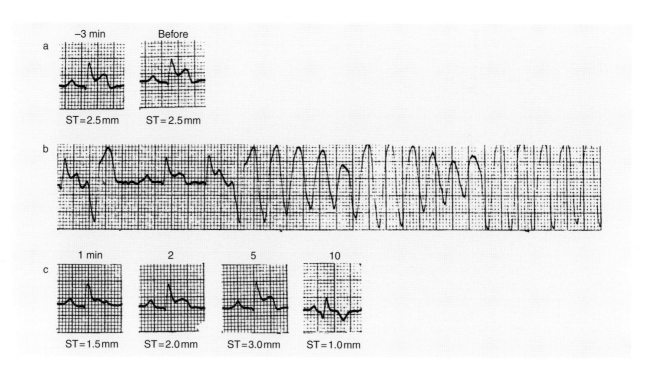

Figure 6.8 *Ischaemia Grade 3 in the pre-infarct syndrome. (a) In the first tracing, the ST segment elevation is 2.5 mm. In (b), note the appearance of an extrasystole after the T waves, and the subsequent polymorphous ventricular tachycardia. The QRS complexes are well defined at a rate of 150–250 beats per minute. (c) Over the next ten minutes, the ST-segment elevation resolved and the T waves became inverted (reperfusion arrhythmia).*

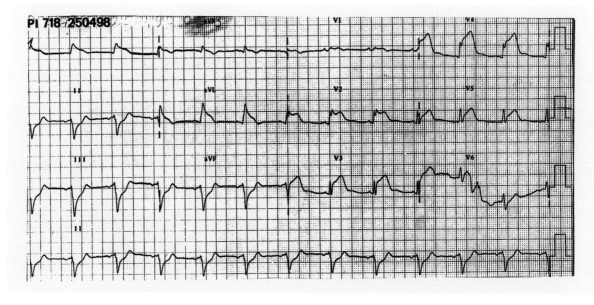

Figure 6.9 *Reperfusion polymorphous ventricular tachycardia. (a) A patient with anterior infarction with ischaemia Grade 3. (b) Twenty minutes after the initiation of thrombolytic therapy, the sinus beats have ECG evidence supporting reperfusion. (c) Polymorphous ventricular tachycardia occurred immediately after this, requiring electrical cardioversion. (d) Note that the beats after cardioversion continue to show signs of reperfusion.*

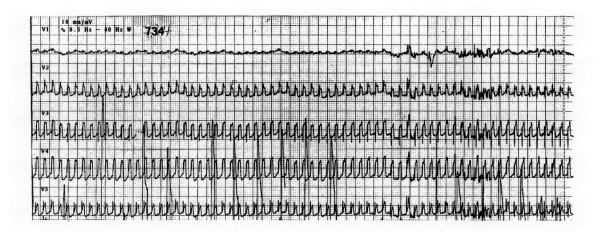

b

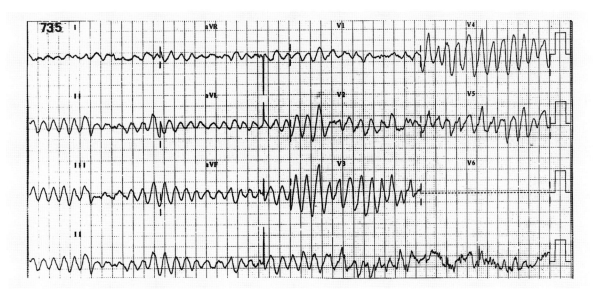

c

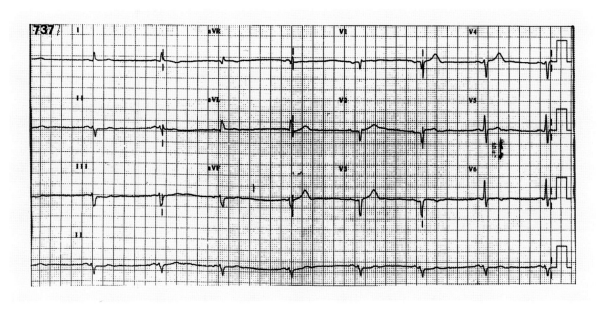

d

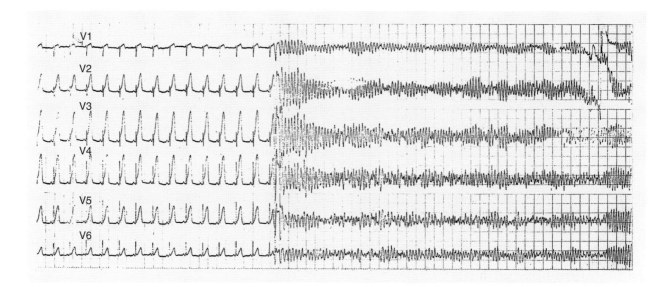

Figure 6.10 *Continuous six-channel ECG recording from a patient with pre-infarct syndrome. During reperfusion, polymorphous ventricular tachycardia occurred (*torsade de pointes *morphology).*

Polymorphous ventricular tachycardia due to reperfusion is a benign manifestation when seen in the coronary care unit but it may end with sudden death in the absence of adequate facilities. These arrhythmias should be reverted with very low electrical energy (100 Joules) or chest percussion.

ACCELERATED IDIOVENTRICULAR RHYTHM

These arrhythmias can be seen in the early stages of reperfusion. They appear even before any signs of reperfusion have been recorded by the ECG, that is

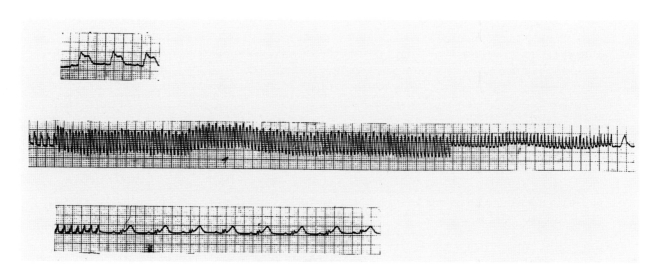

Figure 6.11 *The top panel exhibits ischaemia Grade 3 during pre-infarct syndrome. The middle panel demonstrates the fast ventricular dysrhythmia with* torsade de pointes *morphology (recorded at 5 mm/sec). Note the spontaneous resolution of the tachycardia and the resolution of ST segment elevation immediately after the termination of the tachycardia.*

when there is no evidence of resolution of the ST segment and T wave elevation. They only occur in patients receiving thrombolytic therapy or primary angioplasty. The characteristics of these arrhythmias are:

- the absence of ECG signs of reperfusion;
- a rate similar to the sinus rhythm rate;
- a morphology that varies with the location of the ischaemia.

In the anterior wall ischaemias, the pattern resembles posterior hemiblock. In inferior wall ischaemias, a left anterior hemiblock pattern is seen. During left ventricular ischaemia, these patterns accompany an RBBB-like pattern. Therefore it is of the utmost importance to avoid confusing this morphology with the intermittent right branch blocks that can occur during the ischaemic process (*Fig. 6.12*).

The arrhythmia is not necessarily followed by effective reperfusion as indicated by a significant decrement in the amplitude of ST segment and the T waves. This type of arrhythmia may be induced by non-significant reperfusion in the ischaemic area or by reperfusion in marginal areas, but not by reperfusion in the core of the ischaemia (*Figs 6.13* and *6.14*).

ARRHYTHMIAS IN Q WAVE INFARCTION

No severe arrhythmias are observed at the stage when Q waves have already developed. The most frequent ventricular arrhythmias are:

- extrasystole;
- accelerated idioventricular arrhythmia;
- slow ventricular tachycardia.

Ventricular extrasystoles show non-fixed and large coupling and have a variable morphology. These extrasystoles have a very different pathophysiological mechanism from those discussed above. They arise from the Purkinje system of the ischaemic area as an automatic focus, and therefore they can have different morphologies. An anterior infarct that extends into the lateral, inferior wall and to the right wall of the ventricular septum may cause extrasystoles with an RBBB (left ventricle) pattern with either left axis deviation (inferior wall) or right deviation (anterior wall). The RBBB pattern of the extrasystoles may also manifest as QS waves from leads V2–V6 and qR waves in lead AVR (apex of the interior wall). This infarction may also induce extrasystoles with LBBB

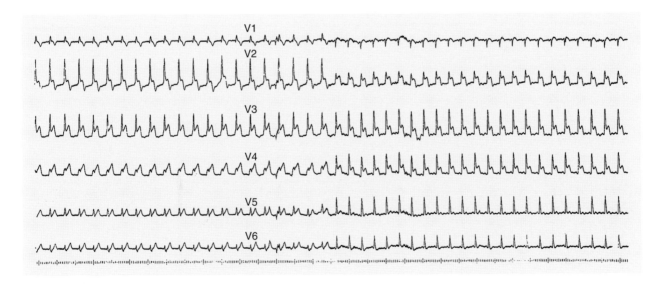

Figure 6.12 *A patient with anterior wall infarction. The first 21 beats are accelerated idioventricular rhythm with an RBBB-like pattern in the very early stage of reperfusion. Thereafter, normal sinus rhythm is resumed. In leads V2–V4 there are still no ECG signs of reperfusion. Note that the heart rate is almost constant during the transition from the idioventricular rhythm to the sinus rhythm, underscoring the fact that this rhythm may go unnoticed or may be erroneously diagnosed as sinus rhythm with transient RBBB.*

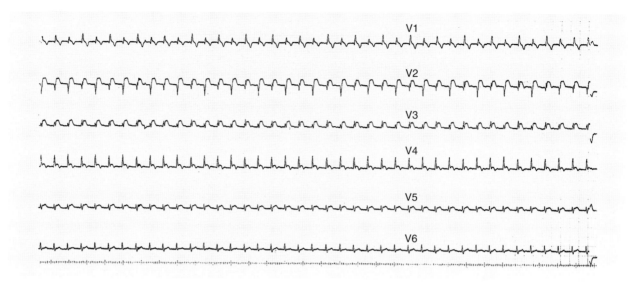

Figure 6.13 *ECG tracing from the same patient as in Fig. 6.12. There is a transient RBBB-like pattern during an idioventricular dysrhythmia. The pattern in the tracings is shorter; this is a fusion beat of the left and right foci.*

and right axis deviation (right ventricle, anterior wall). In spite of the multifocal ventricular arrhythmia and non-fixed coupling, the prognosis is usually benign and malignant arrhythmias do not develop (*Fig. 6.15*).

ACCELERATED IDIOVENTRICULAR RHYTHM DURING REPERFUSION Q WAVE INFARCTION

These arrhythmias have three typical ECG characteristics (*Fig. 6.16*):

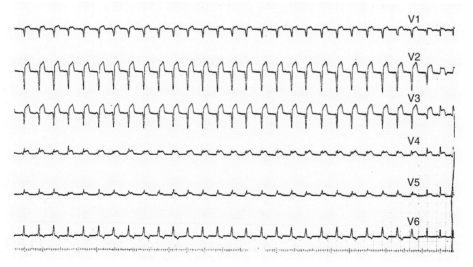

Figure 6.14 *ECG tracing from the same patient as in Figs 6.10 and 6.11. The patient developed idioventricular rhythm with an LBBB-like pattern. The focus is the right side of the septum. The final beats in the tracing are sinus beats. This pattern must be differentiated from intermittent LBBB.*

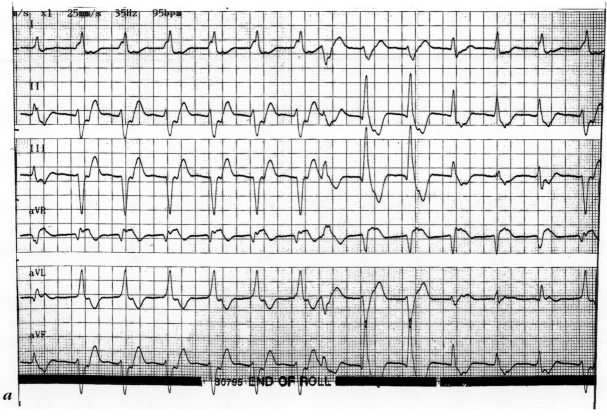

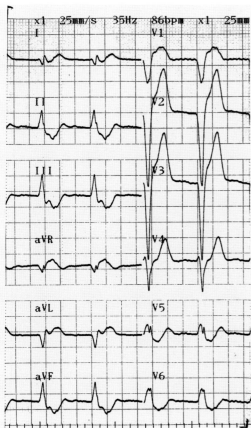

Figure 6.15 *(a) The AIVR was obtained by a 6-lead simultaneous recording in the reperfusion phase of the acute anterior wall infarction. The first beat is a fusion ventricular beat, the next six beats show a ventricular rhythm (98 bpm) with a pattern of extreme left axis deviation (AVR suggest left ventricle origin); the origin of the ventricular rhythm is the posterior wall of the left ventricle. Beats 9–10 show a ventricular rhythm with extreme right axis deviation; AVR suggests right ventricle origin with 90 bpm. Beats 12–14 show no axis deviation; AVR suggests left ventricle origin. The focus of the arrhythmia may be located in the lateral wall of the left ventricle.*

(b) The same patient shows another right axis deviation pattern, however the morphology is different from the previous tracing. Beats 9–10 suggest a different focus of ventricular rhythm in the anterior wall of the right ventricle.

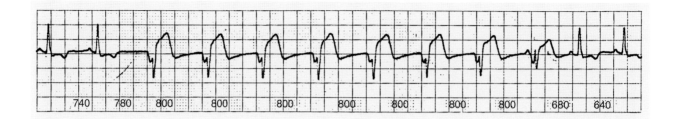

Figure 6.16 *Typical ECG tracings of accelerated idioventricular rhythm. The first two beats show signs of reperfusion (i.e. isoelectric ST segment with inverted T waves). The third beat is a ventricular escape beat. The next six beats are regular ventricular rhythm (interval of 800 msec). The next beat is a fusion beat of sinus origin and ventricular origin. The last two beats are accelerated sinus beats.*

- they start with an escape beat or a late coupling systole;
- the ventricular rhythm is generally regular, with a rate of 60–120 beats per minute;
- the arrhythmia is interrupted by a competitive rhythm (sinus rhythm or a ventricular rhythm).[7]

These arrhythmias appear frequently during the advanced stages of reperfusion when there are inverted T waves and an isoelectric or slightly ele-vated ST segment. The morphology of accelerated idioventricular rhythm depends on the location of the infarcts. In infarcts of the inferior wall there is left axis deviation (*Fig. 6.17*), whereas infarcts of the anterior wall cause right axis deviation (*Fig. 6.18*). In the precordial leads, the morphology of the ventricular arrhythmia may be that of either RBBB or LBBB (*Fig. 6.19*). This is the unique clinical situation where the two foci act in unison conceding a special characteristic to the arrhythmia. In the presence of

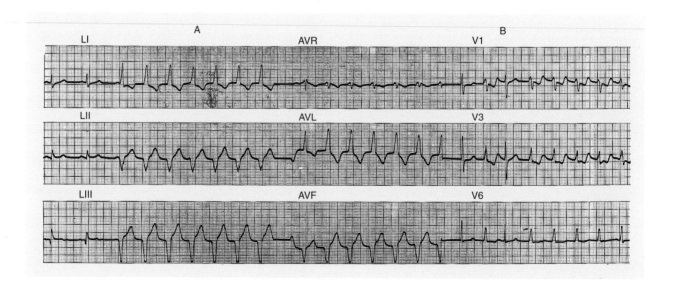

Figure 6.17 *Inferior wall infarction with ECG signs of reperfusion. The first two beats are sinus beats followed by an escape beat and then an idioventricular rhythm. This is the typical evolution of idioventricular rhythm. The morphology of the rhythm is extreme left axis deviation (R wave in leads LI and AVL, and QS in the inferior leads). In leads V2 and V3 the rhythm has an LBBB-like pattern. This morphology suggests that the origin is from the inferior wall and right ventricle.*

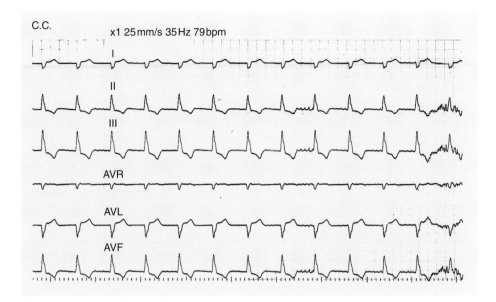

Figure 6.18 *ECG showing accelerated idioventricular rhythm in the patient as in Figs 6.12, 6.13, and 6.14. The rhythm in the standard leads has extreme right axis deviation (QS in leads LI and AVL, and R wave in the inferior leads). The morphology in lead AVR resembles an LBBB-like pattern, suggesting a right anterior origin.*

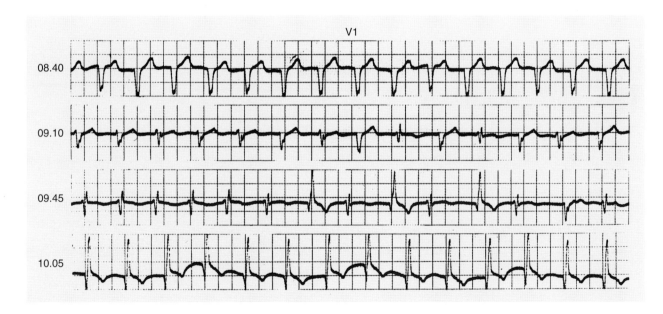

Figure 6.19 *Serial ECG tracings in lead V1 in a patient with inferior wall infarction. The phenomenon illustrated here is unique to accelerated idioventricular rhythm. The top panel demonstrates idioventricular rhythm with an LBBB-like pattern. The second panel has a narrow QRS with a variable morphology, caused by the simultaneous firing from two foci of the same frequency, one in the left side and the other in the right side. The third panel also presents fusion beats with an RBBB-like pattern, although with a narrow QRS, and in between are three beats with a complete RBBB-like pattern. The last panel depicts only the left ventricular focus, again with an RBBB-like pattern. Note that the top and bottom panels have the same heart rate, despite the different morphologies and foci.*

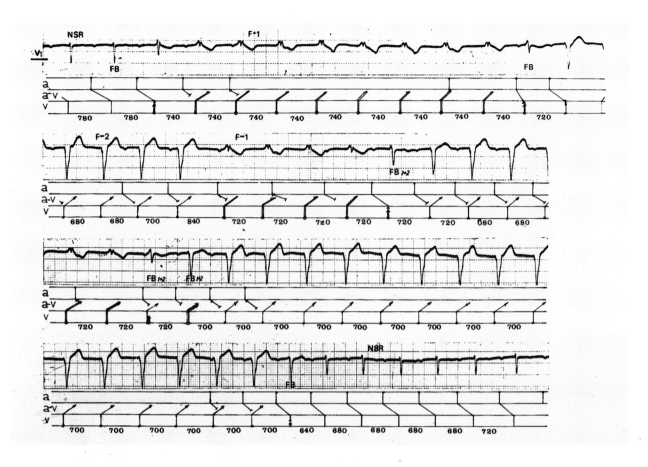

Figure 6.20 *Another patient with two foci of accelerated idioventricular rhythm. In the top panel, there is an RBBB-like pattern, indicating a focus from the left side of the septum. In the second-last beat, there is a fusion beat from the two foci on both sides of the septum. Thereafter, idioventricular rhythm with an LBBB-like pattern developed. During the ensuing beats, there are repeated fusion beats from both foci. The fusion beats are narrower than the other complexes owing to the stimulation from both sides of the septum.*

two foci in two different ventricles and with a similar rate, fusion beats are seen (see *Fig. 6.19*). The fusion beats of two different ventricles hold an intermediate pattern as well as a fusion beat between two foci with different axis (*Figs 6.19* and *6.20*).

Anterior wall infarcts may involve a very extensive area, including the anteroseptal area, anterolateral, inferior wall, and right septum. In this case, it is possible to record four or five different foci of accelerated idioventricular rhythm.[8]

Multifocal ventricular rhythms have a bad prognosis in patients both with and without cardiac pathology, though multifocal accelerated ventricular rhythm appearing during reperfusion in a Q wave infarction is benign and has a good prognosis. These

arrhythmias may persist for hours or days. They are probably autonomous foci induced by the metabolic changes caused by reperfusion.

Inverted T waves indicate that potassium and calcium ions are being washed out from the ischaemic area. These electrolytes thoroughly wash out the Purkinje system, thus inducing arrhythmias of slow current. This assumption may explain the dramatic effect of verapamil on the accelerated idioventricular rhythm; a small dose of intravenous verapamil (1–3 mg) can depress or abolish the foci. These arrhythmias disappear when acute re-ischaemias occur or when the reperfusion process is concluded. As has been stressed in Chapter 4, reperfusion may last up to 72 hours (*Figs 6.21* and *6.22*).

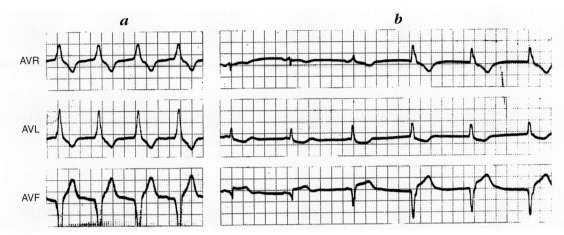

Figure 6.21 *Accelerated idioventricular rhythm during an advanced stage of reperfusion. (a) In lead AVR there is an RBBB-like pattern (left ventricular origin). There is extreme left axis deviation. The heart rate is 80 beats per minute. (b) After the intravenous administration of 2 mg verapamil (a), the rhythm decreased to 56 beats per minute.*

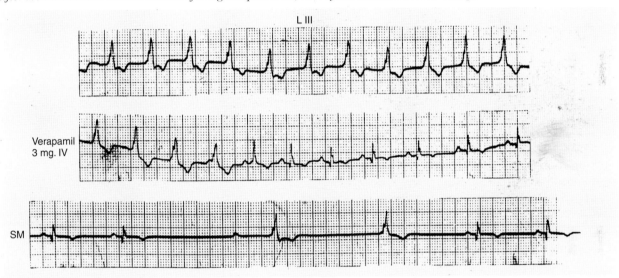

Figure 6.22 *Accelerated idioventricular rhythm in the upper panel in a patient with inferior wall infarction. The heart rate is 100 beats per minute. After the intravenous administration of 3 mg verapamil, the rhythm was completely abolished. The bottom tracing shows that during sinus carotis massage (SM) and reduced sinus frequency, no accelerated idioventricular rhythm could elicited. Note, the same ventricular beats (3 and 4) have the same morphology however, with very low frequency (38bpm).*

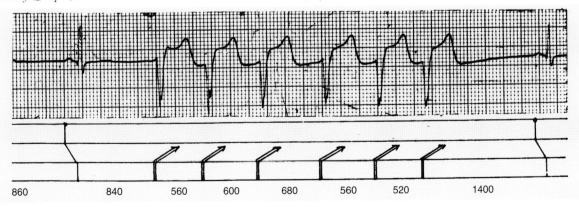

Figure 6.23 *Slow ventricular tachycardia beginning with a late extrasystole and a regular R–R interval, culminating with an exit block.*

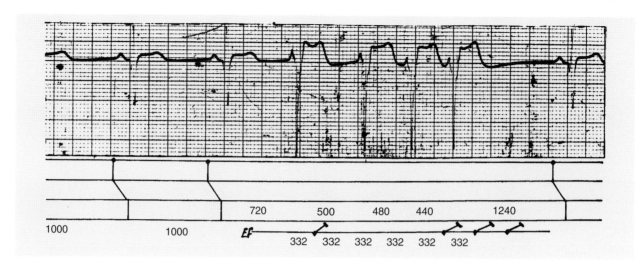

Figure 6.24 *A bout of slow ventricular ventricular tachycardia.*

Non-reperfusion Q wave infarcts do not induce arrhythmias in the first few days. Most ventricular arrhythmias are seen during reperfusion, because in the absence of myocardial reperfusion, no conditions are created for the appearance of arrhythmias. Non-reperfusion Q-wave infarcts usually cause problems from the 15th day onward, with ventricular tachycardia being caused by re-entry; most patients have positive late potentials. Arrhythmias that are observed in these patients are slow ventricular arrhythmias that are characterized by *(Figs 6.23 and 6.24)*:

- onset with early extrasystole;
- irregular rhythm of variable rate;
- conclude with exit block and appear with normal sinus rhythm.

REFERENCES

1. Edwards G, Weston AM. Pharmacology of the potassium channel openers. *Cardiovasc Drug Ther* 1995; **9:** 183–93.

2. Batlee WE, Naimi S, Avitall B, et al. Distinctive time course of ventricular vulnerability to fibrillation during coronary occlusion and release. *Am J Cardiol* 1975; **36:** 776–82.

3. Lombardi G, Gallagher J, Gennis P. Outcome of out-hospital cardiac arrest in New York City. The pre-hospital arrest Survival Evaluation (PHASE) Study. *JAMA* 1994; **271:** 678.

4. Sclarovsky S, Strasberg B, Lahav M, et al. Premature ventricular contraction in acute myocardial infarction: correlation between their origin and the location of the infarction. *J Electrocardiol* 1979; **12:** 157–61.

5. Lucas A, Antzelevitch CH. Differences in the electrophysiological response of canine ventricular epicardium and endocardium ischaemia. *Circulation* 1993; **88:** 2903–75.

6. Birnbaum Y, Sclarovsky S, Ben Ami R, et al. Polymorphous ventricular tachycardia early after acute myocardial infarction. *Am J Cardiol* 1993; **71:** 745–9.

7. Sclarovsky S, Strasberg B, Martonovich G, et al. Ventricular rhythms with intermediate rates in acute myocardial infarction. *Chest* 1978; **74:** 180–2.

8. Sclarovsky S, Strasberg B, Fuchs J, et al. Multiform accelerated idioventricular rhythm in acute myocardial infarction: electrocardiographic characteristics and response to Verapamil. *Am J Cardiol* 1983; **57:** 44–7.

Chapter 7 Conduction impairments in acute ischaemic syndromes

SUMMARY

Conduction impairments correlate with the type of ischaemia causing them as well as with their timing after the acute ischaemic event. A conduction defect appearing during the acute event carries a different prognostic significance to those appearing during reperfusion or later on. There are also patterns of acute ischaemia that are more prone to develop conduction defects than others. For example, ischaemia Grade 3 is the most common type of ischaemia associated with conduction defects. Moreover, it is important to differentiate between defects associated with inferoposterior infarcts and those associated with anterior infarcts.

INFEROPOSTERIOR INFARCTS

Blocks that appear during inferoposterior infarcts are due to altered conduction in the atrioventricular node. Most of them evolve to high-degree atrioventricular blocks. There are two subgroups:[1]

- blocks appearing during the pre-infarct syndrome—these are early blocks or 'ischaemic blocks';[1]
- blocks appearing after an established infarction, usually during the reperfusion phase of Q wave infarction—these are late blocks or 'metabolic blocks'.

EARLY BLOCKS (ISCHAEMIC BLOCKS)

The ECG characteristics of these blocks (*Fig. 7.1*) are as follows:

- they appear in pre-infarct syndrome, and usually disappear with effective reperfusion (*Fig. 7.2*);

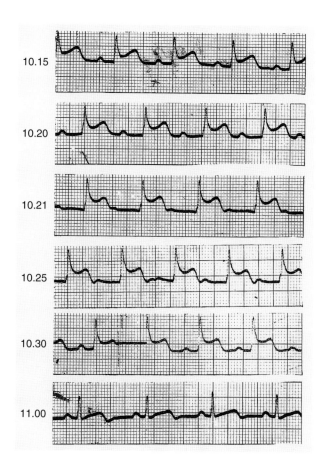

Figure 7.1 *Typical characteristics of early blocks (ischaemic blocks). In the top panel, first-degree atrioventricular block is evident. After 5 minutes (panels 2 and 3), there is a gradual increase in the severity of the block concomitant with the increase in severity of ischaemia. Thereafter, the ischaemia gradually resolves (with signs of reperfusion), as does the degree of atrioventricular block. In the bottom panel, there are signs of complete reperfusion without any evidence of atrioventricular block.*

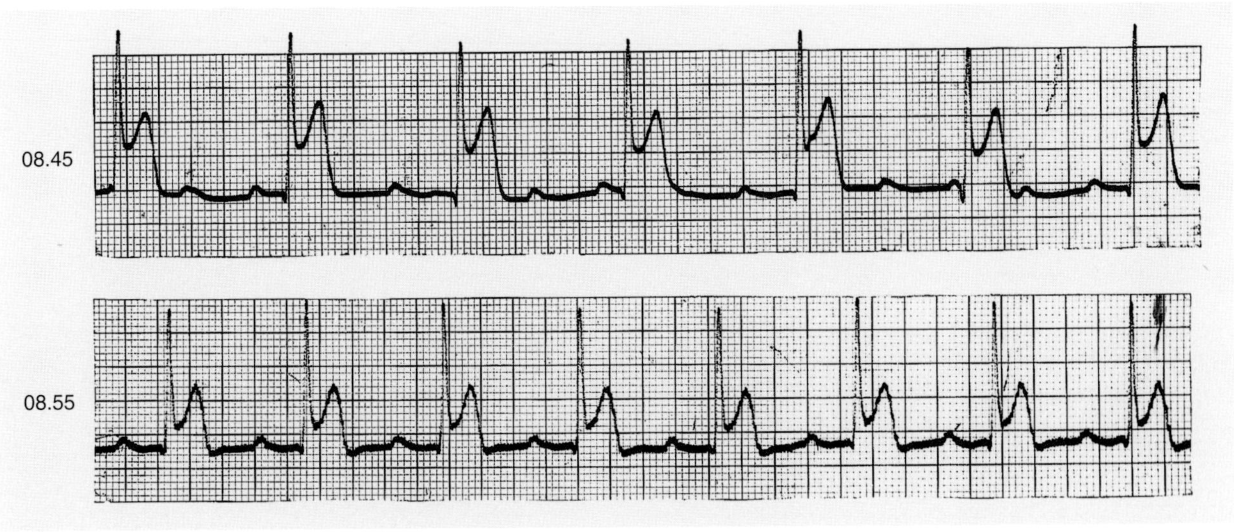

Figure 7.2 *ECG tracings showing the correlation between the acute ischaemic syndrome and atrioventricular blocks. The patient had inferior wall pre-infarct syndrome. In the upper panel, the patient had ST segment elevation of 8 mm and complete atrioventricular block. In the bottom row, the tracing obtained 10 minutes later depicts a lesser amplitude of ST segment elevation and the partial resolution of the block (first-degree block).*

- they appear and disappear acutely (*Fig. 7.3*);
- they may appear as first-degree atrioventricular block, typical or atypical Wenkebach (Mobitz type 1), Mobitz type 2, or even third-degree atrioventricular block (*Fig. 7.4*);
- the grade of ischaemia is usually Grade 3 (see *Fig. 7.3*).[2]

Most of these blocks are accompanied by right ventricular infarctions.[3] They are associated with higher rates of mortality and morbidity than infarcts without blocks.[1] At times, a temporary pacemaker may be needed to preserve the haemodynamic status.[1]

The mechanism for these blocks may be anatomical or biochemical.

Blocks caused by anatomical abnormalities

The atrioventricular branch arises from the posterior descending coronary artery (a branch of the right coronary artery in 90% of people).[4] Most of these blocks occur in patients with obstructions in the artery proximal to the origin of the atrioventricular

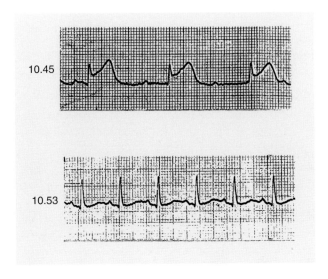

Figure 7.3 *Inferior wall pre-infarct syndrome with complete atrioventricular block in lead LII. Eight minutes later, there were ECG signs of reperfusion with resolution of the block.*

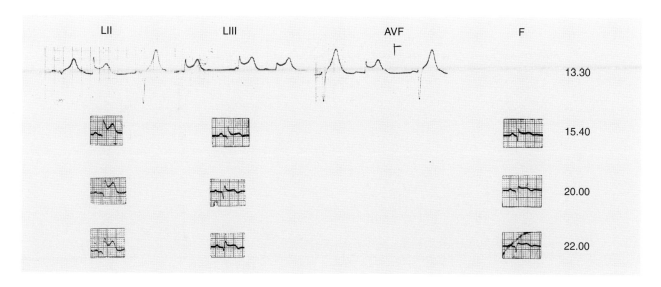

Figure 7.4 *The upper panel exhibits ECG tracings obtained at the patient's home 40 minutes after the onset of chest pain. There is severe sinus bradycardia. The third beat in lead LIII depicts a prolonged PR interval. At 15.40 the patient was admitted to the coronary care unit with persistent symptoms and first-degree block (a PR interval of 220 msec). During reperfusion, the PR interval returned to normal.*

branch. This also explains the high rate of right ventricular infarctions associated with these blocks.

Blocks caused by biochemical abnormalities

During the acute ischaemic episode, adenosine is released into the infarcted areas as the result of accelerated degradation of ATP. The sinus node and the atrioventricular node have adenosine receptors (A2 receptors).[5] Stimulation of these receptors produces a negative chronotropic and dromotropic effect. This may be a protective mechanism whereby oxygen consumption is reduced. However, this may prove to be detrimental when there is haemodynamic compromise.

Interestingly, during an attempt to block the effect of adenosine during these conduction impairments using the adenosine antagonist aminophylline,[6] it was not possible to prevent the reverse of these blocks. Thus it seems that the anatomical explanation is of greater significance. Supporting this contention is the fact that upon reperfusion, these blocks often disappear acutely.

These blocks may reappear upon re-ischaemic events (*Fig. 7.5*). Thus, the author prefers to refer to them as ischaemic blocks. During the appearance of these blocks, the myocardium is highly susceptible to ventricular arrhythmias. We have shown that an electrode in contact with right ventricle during these blocks may cause lethal ventricular fibrillation. Likewise, during manipulation in the catheterization laboratory, lethal arrhythmias may arise in these patients.[7]

LATE BLOCKS (METABOLIC BLOCKS)

These blocks have distinct ECG characteristics[1]:

- they usually appear 24 hours after the onset of the acute event, although in some patients this develops during the first 12 hours (*Fig. 7.6*);
- they are usually associated with ECG signs of reperfusion;
- the block is usually a typical Wenkebach-type block (Mobitz type 1);
- the evolution and disappearance are gradual (over 24–36 hours).

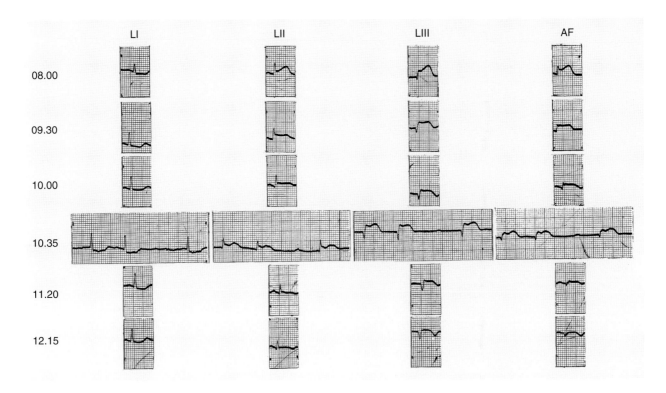

Figure 7.5 *At 08.00 (top panel) the patient had inferior wall pre-infarct syndrome with ischaemia Grade 3 in lead AVF. At this stage, the patient did not have an atrioventricular block. The second and third panels depict ECG signs of reperfusion. At 10.35 (fourth panel) there was re-ischaemia with evidence of sinus bradycardia and atypical high-degree atrioventricular block. The last two panels depict signs of reperfusion and normalization of conduction. This case demonstrates that atrioventricular blocks may appear during the re-ischaemic events rather than during the initial episode.*

Usually a late block begins with first-degree atrioventricular block. First, the PR interval is prolonged to 240–260 msec, and then Wenkebach blocks appear. This is usually 5:4 at first, progressing to 3:2. If progression continues, complete atrioventricular block may occur with an escape rhythm from the nodal origin of 45–60 beats/minute. The recovery phase is a mirror image of the first phase. The first-degree atrioventricular block may last up to 10 days. The Wenkebach block usually lasts between 1 and 5 days. The prognosis of patients with late blocks resembles that of the patients without late blocks.[1]

Temporary pacing is rarely needed in this type of block, as opposed to the early blocks. The author, with over 28 years' experience, can recall only one patient in whom a permanent pacemaker was needed after developing a late block.

The aetiology of these blocks may be the release of potassium and calcium during the reperfusion process or during myocyte necrosis. This, along with the cholinergic excitation, produces a considerable depression of conduction.[8] The maximal efflux of potassium and calcium is after the first 24 hours. The duration of the block is most probably dependent on the washout of these metabolites. Thus, the author refers to these blocks as 'metabolic blocks'. Interestingly, these blocks may respond to atropine, which accelerates the nodal rhythm to 70 beats/minute. This is achieved by blocking the cholinergic contribution.

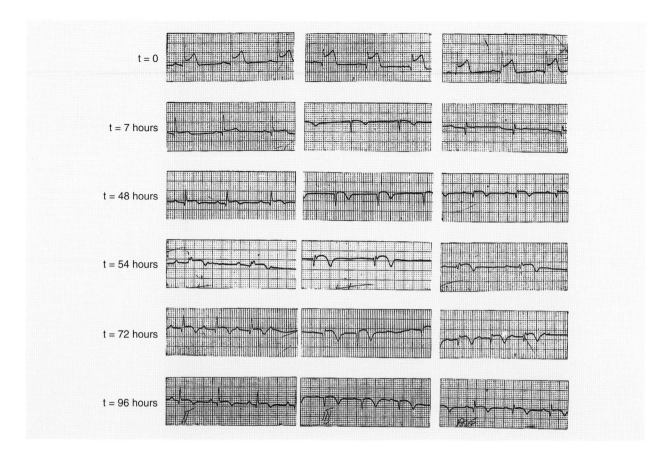

t = 0

t = 7 hours

t = 48 hours

t = 54 hours

t = 72 hours

t = 96 hours

Figure 7.6 *ECG tracings showing typical late block (metabolic block). In the top panel, inferior wall pre-infarct syndrome is evident in leads LII, LIII, and AVF. There are no signs of atrioventricular conduction defects. Seven hours later (second panel), complete reperfusion is evident, predominantly in lead LIII. There are still no conduction defects. Forty-eight hours later (third panel), there are no signs of re-ischaemia. Nevertheless, the PR interval is prolonged. One day later (fifth panel), high-degree atrioventricular block developed, with a gradual resolution over the next 24 hours until its complete disappearance the next day (bottom panel).*

ATYPICAL BLOCKS DURING INFEROPOSTERIOR INFARCTS

The most common atypical block in inferoposterior infarcts is the Wenkebach block with alternate beats. Less well known is longitudinal dissociation of the atrioventricular node.

Wenkebach block with alternate beats

In order to understand the Wenkebach block with alternate beats (*Fig. 7.7*), it is important to review the structure of the atrioventricular node. This node is composed of three components, each with distinct electrophysiological attributes. The upper part (AN) is in contact with the lower right atrium. The middle part (N) is above the lower part (NH).

AN possess two properties:[9]

- the ability to maintain the heart rate at 50 beats/minute;
- electrotonic augmentation, unlike the decremental conduction that is below the atrioventricular system.[11]

The nodal rhythm is under the control of neuroregulation. Like the sinus node, this node is depressed by cholinergic stimulation, although it is

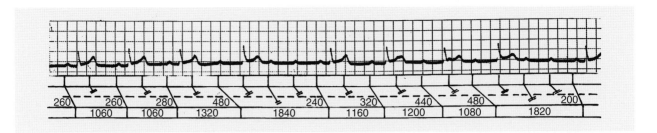

Figure 7.7 *ECG tracing of atrioventricular block with alternate Wenkebach beats. The ladder under the tracing demonstrates that the first beat has a prolonged PR interval (260 msec). The next beat is dropped. This is followed by a beat with a PR interval of 260 msec followed by a dropped beat. The fifth beat has a PR interval of 280 msec. The sixth beat is blocked again. The next beat has a PR interval of 480 msec, followed by three consecutive dropped beats. Thereafter, this phenomenon is repeated.*

less sensitive than the sinus node. The typical ischaemic and metabolic blocks occur at AN in the upper layers.[10,11] In contrast, during these atypical blocks, the blocks are at two levels: at the AN level, and at the N level.

The conduction in these blocks is very slow, and may even degenerate to paroxysmal block with arrest, as in interventricular block. In the typical Wenkebach rhythm there is a progressive prolongation of the PR interval, although each P wave is followed by an R wave. The R–R interval shortens as does the RP interval. There is a drop beat when the P is not followed by a QRS complex. The next sinus beat is conducted normally.

In Wenkebach of alternating beats, there are two P waves in each R–R segment; the first one is not conducted whereas the second P wave is conducted aberrantly, with Wenkebach conduction (see *Fig. 7.12*). Before the dropped beat there are three consecutive P waves. The third P wave is conducted normally (*Figs 7.7* and *7.8*).

These blocks are called transverse blocks and were first described by others as two loci in the intraventricular conduction system with a block (in the infra-His system) (*Fig. 7.9*).[12] However, the author and co-workers have demonstrated clinically that this block is within the atrioventricular node during the inferoposterior infarction.[13]

Atropine may be detrimental, because it improves conduction at AN but not N, thus possibly causing cardiac arrest. Temporary pacing is highly recommended (*Fig. 7.10*).[14]

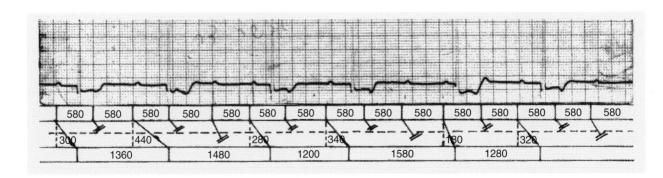

Figure 7.8 *ECG tracing of atrioventricular block with alternate Wenkebach beats.*

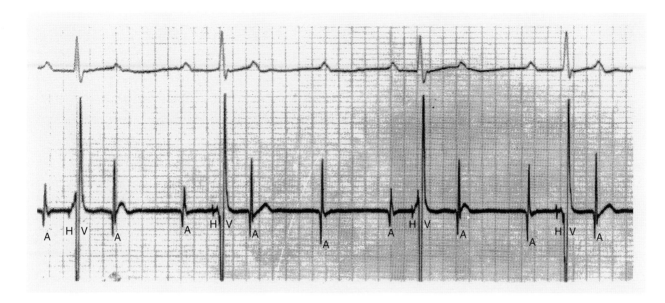

Figure 7.9 *Typical atrioventricular block with alternate Wenkebach beats, with simultaneous His-bundle recording. Note that the blocked A wave is supra-His. The conducted beats have an H wave before the V wave. A, atrim; H, His; V, ventricle.*

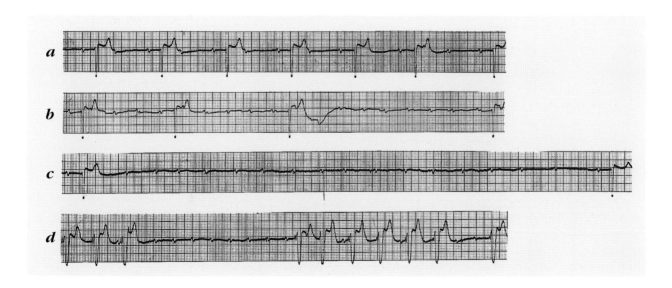

Figure 7.10 *The top panel (a) depicts typical characteristics of Wenkebach of alternate beats. In (b), paroxysmal atrioventricular block can be seen accompanied by the occurrence of syncope. In (c), after the administration of atropine, the block worsened although the sinus rhythm was accelerated. In (d), a temporary pacemaker was inserted.*

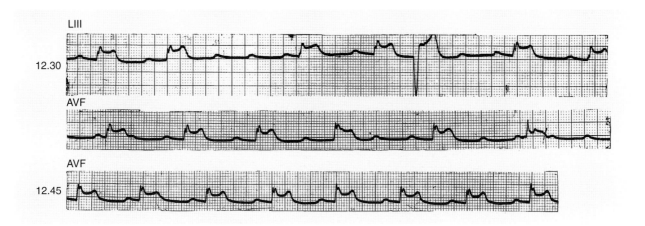

Figure 7.11 *In the top two panels, the ECG illustrates inferior wall pre-infarct syndrome in leads LIII and AVF with alternate Wenkebach beats during the pre-infarct syndrome. Fifteen minutes later there were ECG signs of reperfusion, and the bottom panel depicts the disappearance of the block with a residual first degree atrioventricular block (PR of 320 msec).*

Most of these blocks occur early (*Fig. 7.11*), although at times they may also appear in later stages. The presence of these blocks portends a poor prognosis because of the haemodynamic compromise associated with these conduction impairments.

Longitudinal dissociation of the atrioventricular node

This phenomenon is well known among electro-physiologists, although it is not often related to acute ischaemia.[15] However, acute ischaemic syndrome can produce this phenomenon.[16]

In this impairment, there are two intranodal anterograde pathways with different refractory times and conduction velocities. This is recognized by the appearance of two different PR intervals and is evident either in the pre-infarct stage or later on (*Figs 7.12* and *7.13*). It disappears after several days, usually spontaneously, and it bears a benign prognosis. It usually does not recur, attesting to its link to the ischaemic process. During the acute episode, each pathway may be unveiled by blocking the other with an extrasystole.

ANTERIOR INFARCTS

Atrioventricular blocks during anterior wall infarction are fortunately uncommon. The most common manifestation is bifascicular block. Right bundle branch block (RBBB) with or without blocks in the left fascicle does often occur in transmural regional ischaemic syndrome. However, because RBBB is common among the general population, pre-existing blocks must be differentiated from new blocks.

Right bundle branch block and left anterior hemiblock (LAHB) frequently occur together because of a common anatomic defect, that is the impaired blood supply by the septal branches of the left anterior descending coronary artery.[17] It is important to distinguish between these blocks occurring during the pre-infarct syndrome from those occurring later on. Most of these blocks are transient. When these blocks occur during the pre-infarct syndrome, they have the following characteristics (*Figs 7.14* and *7.15*):

- they occur when there is maximal ST segment elevation with upright T waves;
- most disappear upon the appearance of reperfusion in the ECG.

Thus, this is an ischaemic block in anterior infarcts. Most of these patients have a lesion in the proximal left anterior descending coronary artery.

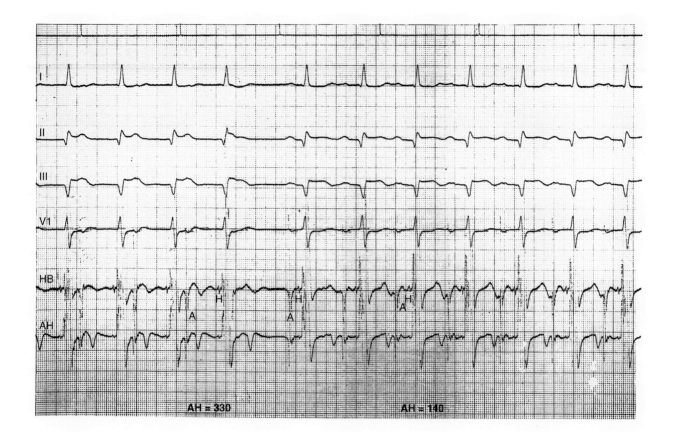

Figure 7.12 *Longitudinal dissociation of the atrioventricular node during inferior wall infarction. The upper three rows demonstrate the typical pattern of inferior wall pre-infarct syndrome. The last two rows demonstrate simultaneous His recordings. In lead V1, P waves are evident just before the T waves. Note that the intracardiac recordings demonstrate an atrial spike at the same time interval as the P wave on the ECG. The AH interval (time interval for conduction from atrium to His) is 330 msec. The fifth beat is blocked at the nodal level; the atrial impulse is not propagated. Thereafter, the PR interval is short and the AH interval is 160 msec.*

There is usually ST segment elevation in lead V1 (representing the septal branches supplying the right ventricular portion of the intraventricular septum). It is rare to see this block in anterior pre-infarction syndrome in patients without ST segment elevation in lead V1. If this block does not resolve during reperfusion, it is associated with a poor prognosis (*Fig. 7.16*).

When this block appears in the reperfusion stage or even later, this may represent a leakage of metabolites from myocytes, as described above for metabolic blocks during inferior infarcts[18,19] (*Fig. 7.17*). The prognosis in these cases is usually benign, and the block may resolve on restoration of the metabolite balance (usually within 24 hours). As described above, this block occurring at these later stages is also associated with proximal lesions in the left anterior descending coronary artery (*Figs 7.18, 7.19* and *7.20*).

It is important to differentiate this block from idioventricular rhythms of left ventricular origin with a right bundle branch block-like pattern. When this block is persistent, the prognosis is ominous owing to the extensive structural damage, and also to the conduction damage.

A unique situation occurs when there is LAHB

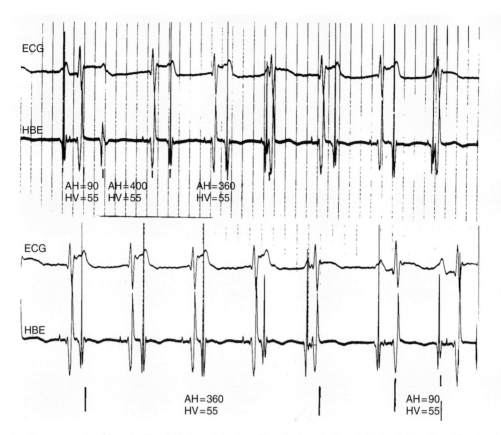

Figure 7.13 *Another example of longitudinal atrioventricular dissociation during inferior infarction. The first beat has an AH interval (time interval for conduction from His to ventricle) of 90 msec. The second beat is an atrial extrasystole with an AH interval of 400 msec. Subsequent beats have an AH interval of 300 msec. In the fifth beat, the blocked atrial spike was seen. The last two beats have a normal PR interval.*

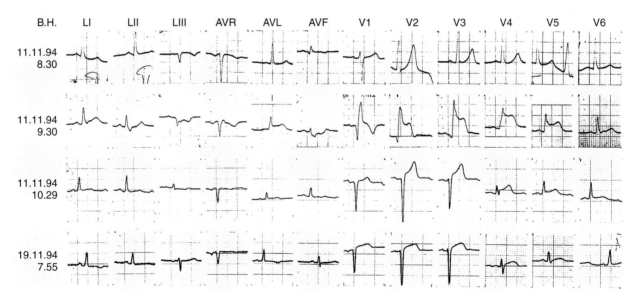

Figure 7.14 *A typical case of ischaemic RBBB in a patient with anterior wall pre-infarct syndrome. In the top panel, the tracing was obtained shortly after a bout of chest pain. One hour later (second panel), the pre-infarct syndrome was evident with the new appearance of RBBB. Note the marked ST segment elevation in lead V1. One hour later (third panel), signs of incomplete reperfusion were noted, and the block disappeared permanently.*

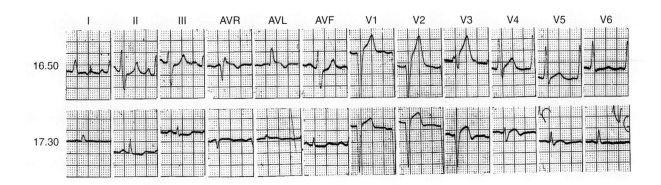

Figure 7.15 *ECG tracings show wide left anterior hemiblock (masking RBBB) in anterior wall infarction. Note the marked ST segment elevation in lead V1 and upright T waves. The R' in lead AVR and the wide S wave in leads V5 and V6 suggest the existence of RBBB. The bottom panel demonstrates the disappearance of the block with the appearance of reperfusion.*

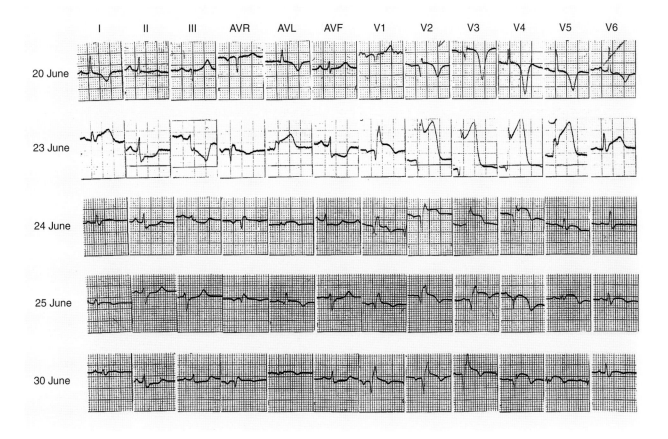

Figure 7.16 *The top panel shows Q wave of reperfusion during infarction. Three days later (second panel), signs of reinfarction were noted, along with the new appearance of RBBB. Note the ST segment elevation in lead V1. Over the next 7 days, signs of extensive anterior wall infarction were evident without resolution of the block.*

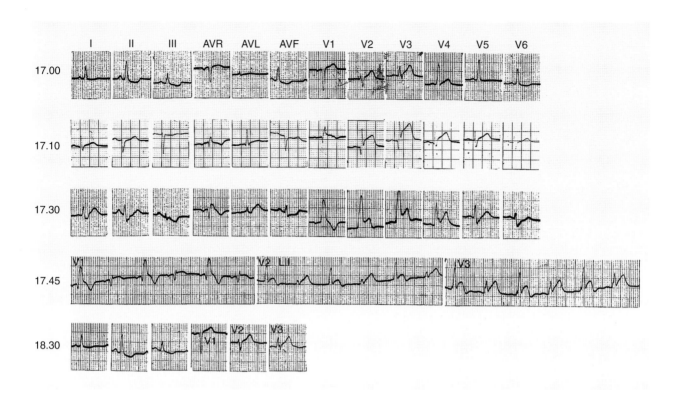

Figure 7.17 *In the upper panel, the tracing depicts anterior wall pre-infarct syndrome without any indication of conduction blocks. Note the ST segment elevation in lead V1. The second panel shows that the ischaemia has spread to leads V2 and V3. There is a concomitant incomplete RBBB with left axis deviation. Twenty minutes later (third panel) the ST segment elevation has partially resolved, but complete RBBB has developed without left axis deviation. In the fourth panel, there is additional resolution of the ST segment elevation and intermittent RBBB. The first three beats in the bottom panel are from leads LI, LII, LIII respectively and the last three beats are from leads V1, V2, and V3. The morphology of the QRS resembles that of the top panel, but there are no signs of block. This case demonstrates that the block appears and is exacerbated in the very early stage of reperfusion. Note that in the bottom panel the ECG morphology (LI, LII, LIII, V1–V3) is similar to the upper panel, indicating that the block was a transient ischaemic block that resolved after reperfusion.*

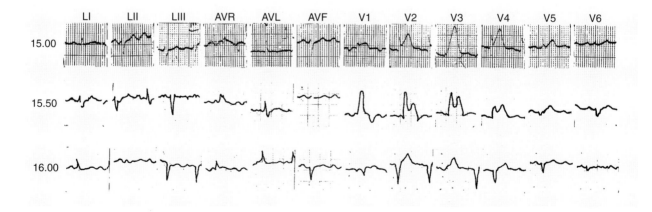

Figure 7.18 *The top panel shows anterior wall pre-infarct syndrome with incomplete RBBB. Note the ST segment elevation in lead V1. Fifty minutes later (second panel) there are signs of reperfusion and the appearance of RBBB, as shown in Figure 7.17. One hour later, there were signs of almost complete reperfusion, and the block disappeared.*

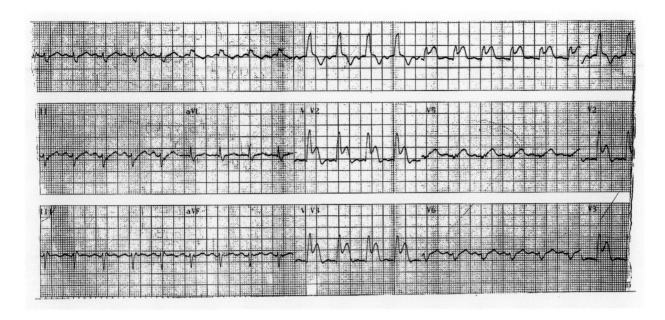

Figure 7.19 *ECG tracings of another case of RBBB and LAHB appearing during the reperfusion stage.*

masquerading as RBBB during anterior infarcts.[20] These blocks have the following characteristics:

- they appear 24 hours after the onset of infarction (*Fig. 7.21*);
- the evolution of the ECG is predictable (*Fig. 7.22*);
- the first aberrance is characteristic LAHB with a narrow QRS complex (*Fig. 7.22*).

Later, there is a progressive widening of the QRS complex in frontal leads (to more than 120 msec). Indirect evidence of RBBB appears, such as wide R' in lead AVR and a wide S in leads V5 and V6. In the ascending limb of the QRS complex in lead 1 there is a notch, but this is evident only when lead V1 is placed a bit higher on the sternum than its usual location (see *Fig. 7.22*). The disappearance of this block is a mirror image of its appearance (see *Fig. 7.22*).

The QRS anomaly may completely resolve or may

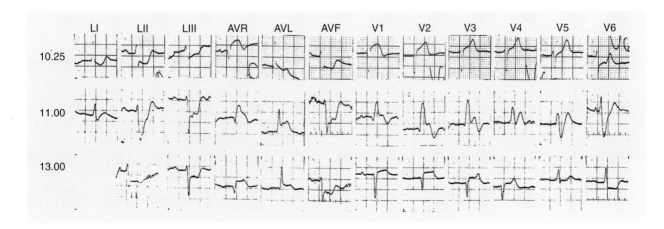

Figure 7.20 *The top panel shows anterior wall pre-infarct syndrome without signs of intraventricular conduction defect. The middle panel shows very wide RBBB with left anterior hemiblock; ECG showing evidence of reperfusion. The bottom panel, recorded two hours later, shows evidence of a first stage of reperfusion and narrow left anterior hemiblock.*

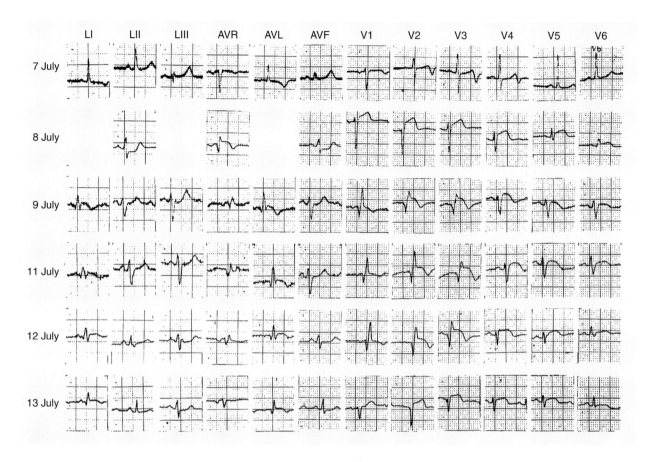

Figure 7.21 *In the top panel there is non-Q wave infarction of the anterior wall. The second row shows re-infarction at which time blocks were not evident. Note the ST segment elevation in lead V1. One day later (second panel), RBBB and LAHB appeared. The LAHB had disappeared by 5 days later (fifth panel) but the RBBB had not. On the sixth day (bottom panel), the RBBB disappeared. This course is typical for metabolic blocks.*

persist as LAHB. Because this is usually a transient block with a predictable course irrespective of recurrent ischaemic events, this is probably a manifestation of metabolic rather than ischaemic processes. Interestingly, this pattern occurs in up to 7–10% of patients with anterior infarcts. Only rarely does this block progress to complete atrioventricular block.

Left bundle branch block may also occur during anterior infarcts. Because this block is common among patients with non-coronary heart disease, such as calcific aortic stenosis or mechanical block,[18] and because it may be intermittent, the acute occurrence of this anomaly must be distinguished from a pre-existing LBBB. In our experience, new LBBB is rare in anterior infarcts. This is because the left bundle branch common trunk is situated in an area of the myocardium that is supplied by a tiny branch arising from the most proximal part of the left anterior descending coronary artery.[19] This artery is very rarely affected during acute ischaemia. In contrast, the anterior and posterior fascicles of the left bundle branch are affected by the individual epicardial circulation. However, because the common trunk is located between the aorta and the mitral valve in a vulnerable, fibrous surrounding,[21] it may be affected by other processes in acute coronary events, such as mechanical stretch during ischaemia.[20]

As explained in Chapter 4, acute LBBB may occur during acute circumferential subendocardial ischaemia, and is usually accompanied by right-axis deviation, perhaps because of traction on the left posterior fascicle during the acute dilatation of the left ventricle (traction block). This is associated with an ominous prognosis (*Fig. 7.23*). In contrast, RBBB and LAHB are rare occurrences during circumferential subendocardial ischaemia.[22]

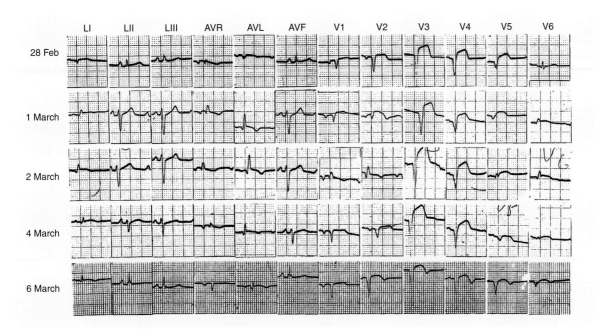

Figure 7.22 *Another case of LAHB with masking RBBB in anterior infarction. The tracing in the top panel was obtained after 24 hours after onset of pain. There were no signs of block. The next day (second panel), extreme LAHB developed. The R' in lead AVR suggests that RBBB may also be present, as does the wide QRS complex (120 msec) in the inferior leads. The third panel shows clearer signs of RBBB. On the fifth day (fourth panel), there is narrow LAHB. Note that the R' in lead AVR has disappeared, as has the wide QRS in leads V1 and V2. The bottom panel shows no signs of block on the seventh day. This is the typical course of metabolic blocks.*

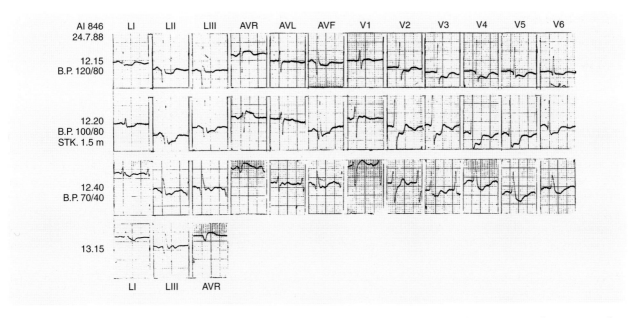

Figure 7.23 *The first panel depicts acute circumferential subendocardial ischaemia. Note the ST segment depression with inverted T waves in leads V3–V5. Five minutes later (second row), a marked depression in the ST segment was evident in leads V2–V5. The axis shifted to the right in the frontal plane. In the third row, signs of left bundle branch block became evident, with widening of the QRS complex and the disappearance of the Q wave in leads V5 and V6. Concomitantly, severe haemodynamic deterioration became evident at 12:40 (20 minutes after the tracing obtained in row 2). The bottom tracing was obtained a few minutes before the patient died.*

REFERENCES

1. Sclarovsky S, Strasberg B, Hirshberg A, et al. Advanced early and late atrioventricular block in acute myocardial infarction. *Am Heart J* 1984; **108:** 19–24.

2. Birnbaum Y, Sclarovsky S, Herz I, et al. Admission clinical and electrocardiographic characteristics predicting in-hospital development of high degree atrioventricular block in inferior wall acute myocardial infarction. *Am J Cardiol* 1997; **80:** 1139–43.

3. Strasberg B, Pinchas A, Arditti A, et al. Left and right ventricular function in inferior acute myocardial infarction and significance of advanced atrioventricular block. *Am J Cardiol* 1984; **54:** 978–85.

4. James TN. The coronary circulation and conduction system in acute myocardial infarction. *Prog Cardiovasc Dis* 1968; **10:** 410.

5. Linden J, Burne R. The cardiac effect of adenosine. *Prog Cardiovasc Dis* 1987; **32:** 73–9.

6. Strasberg B, Bassevich R, Mager A, et al. Effects of aminophylline on atrioventricular conduction in patients with late atrioventricular block during inferior acute myocardial infarction. *Am J Cardiol* 1991; **March 1:** 527–8.

7. Sclarovsky S, Zafrir N, Strasberg B, et al. Ventricular fibrillation complicating temporary ventricular pacing in acute myocardial infarction. Significance of right ventricular infarction. *Am J Cardiol* 1981; **48:** 1160–6.

8. Zipes D. Recent observations supporting the role of slow current in cardiac electrophysiology. In: *Conduction System of the Heart* (Wellens HJJ, Lee KI, Janse MJ, eds). Philadelphia: Lea & Febiger: 1976.

9. Janse M, Van Capelle FJL, Anderson RH, et al. Electrophysiology and structure of the atrioventricular node of the isolated rabbit heart. In: *Conduction System of the Heart* (Wellens, Lee, Janse, eds). Philadelphia: Lea & Febiger: 1976.

10. Mendez C, Mol CK. Some characteristics of transmembrane potential in A-V nodal cell during propagation in premature beats. *Circ Res* 1969; **19:** 993.

11. Janse MJ. Influence of the direction of the atrial wave front on A-V nodal transmission in isolated heart of rabbits. *Circ Res* 1969; **25:** 439.

12. Halpern MS, Naug J, Levi RS, et al. Wenckebach periods in alternate beats. *Circulation* 1973; **48:** 41–9.

13. Sclarovsky S, Lewin R, Strasberg B, et al. Dissociation of the atrioventricular node in acute inferior wall myocardial infarction. 1) Transverse dissociation (alternate Wenckebach periods). *Chest* 1978; **73:** 634–7.

14. Lewin R, Kusniec J, Sclarovsky S, et al. Alternating Wenckebach periods in acute inferior myocardial infarction. Clinical, electrocardiographic and therapeutic characterization. *Pace* 1986; **9:** 468–75.

15. Denes P, Wu D, Dh RC, et al. Dual A-V nodal pathways. *Br Heart J* 1975; **37:** 1069.

16. Sclarovsky S, Lewin R, Strasberg B, et al. Dissociation of the atrioventricular node in acute inferior wall myocardial infarction. 2) Longitudinal dissociation (dual atrioventricular nodal pathways). *Chest* 1978; **73:** 638–41.

17. Ben Gal T, Sclarovsky S, Herz I, et al. The importance of the conal branch of the right coronary artery in patients with acute anterior wall myocardial infarction. *Am J Coll Cardiol* 1997; **29:** 506–11.

18. Wennemarks N, Questa VJ, Brody DA. Microelectrode study of delayed conduction in the canine right bundle branch block. *Circ Res* 1968; **23:** 753–69.

19. Cranefield FP. The conduction of slow response. In: *The Conduction of the Cardiac Impulse.* New York: Futura Publishing: 1975: 115.

20. Sclarovsky S, Lewin R, Strasberg B, et al. Left anterior hemiblock obscuring the diagnosis of right bundle branch block in acute myocardial infarction. *Circulation* 1979; **60:** 26–32.

21. Lenegre J. Etiology and pathology of bilateral bundle branch block in relation to complete heart block. *Prog Cardiovasc Dis* 1964; **6:** 409.

22. Sclarovsky S, Sagie A, Strasberg B, et al. Ischaemic blocks during early phase of anterior infarction: correlation with ST-segment shift. *Clin Cardiol* 1988; **11:** 757–62.

Chapter 8 **Case Studies**

INTRODUCTION

In this chapter we shall analyse the ischaemic process of the anterior wall of the left ventricle. The role of the 'morphological ECG' in cases of chronic ischaemia is important, together with other non-invasive techniques. In acute ischaemia however, the 'morphological ECG' has a pivotal role, dominating all other non-invasive techniques.

In this introduction we want to summarise our hypothesis about the contribution of the ECG to the diagnosis of the acute ischaemic syndrome. The second part of the book analyses the contribution of the ECG in identifying different phases of the ischaemic process provoked by sudden coronary artery obstruction. Chapter 1 discusses the three types of acute ischaemia by a sudden obstruction of a coronary artery:

- acute regional transmural ischaemia;
- acute regional subendocardial ischaemia; and
- acute circumferential ischaemia.

The ECG findings in types 1 and 2 are manifestations of the altered metabolic processes in the ischaemic area. The ECG findings in type 3 result from the sudden increase of the diastolic pressure in the left ventricle during an acute episode. Moreover, the ECG can discriminate between three phases: acute obstruction, reperfusion, and the final outcome, which is responsible for the various myocardial ischaemic syndromes. These syndromes depend in turn on three factors: the obstructed artery, the time of obstruction, and the grade of myocardial protection. The obstructive phase is identified in the acute myocardial ischaemia and the pre-infarction syndrome. The ECG in the obstructive phases provide the following data:

- coronary anatomy:
    (a) culprit artery;
    (b) level of obstruction;
    (c) dimension of the artery.
- myocardial anatomy:
    (a) the core of ischaemia;
    (b) border zone;
    (c) the involvement of the right ventricle.
- ischaemic physiology:
    (a) the grade of ischaemia in each lead;
    (b) the reciprocal phenomenon;
    (c) the attenuation phenomenon.

The following cases are arranged in increasingly more severe manifestations of the acute ischaemic syndrome, ranging from non-Q wave infarction through subendocardial and reperfusion infarction and culminating in non-reperfusion-Q wave infarction.

The relationship between the type of ischaemia due to sudden obstruction of a major coronary artery, the duration of obstruction, and the myocardial consequence of the ischaemic episode (ischaemic myocardial syndrome).

Figures 8.1–8.5 show the relationship between the grade of ischaemia, duration of obstruction and the myocardial ischaemic syndrome in the transmural region ischaemic syndromes.

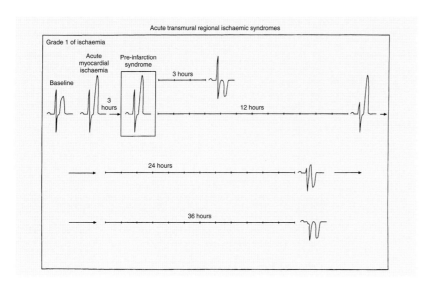

Figure 8.1 *ECG tracings characteristic of ischaemia grade 1, denoting maximal myocardial protection. Reperfusion Q-wave infarction develops only after prolonged obstruction.*

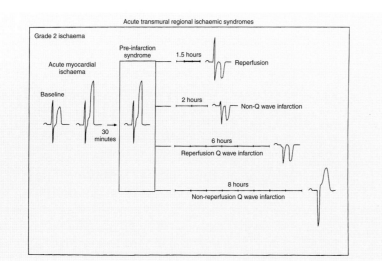

Figure 8.2 *A characteristic ECG tracing of ischaemia grade 2 denoting a moderately-protected heart. This type of ischaemia yields syndromes ranging from non-Q to reperfusion Q-wave infarctions. The window of opportunity to intervene is intermediate between grades 1 and 3 of ischaemia.*

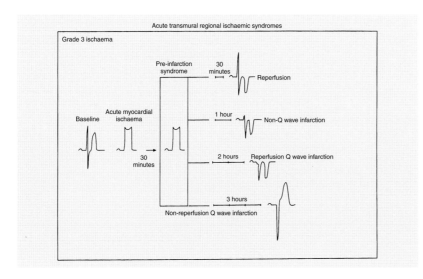

Figure 8.3 *Ischaemia grade 3 denoting a vulnerable myocardium without protection. In this case, reperfusion must be instituted promptly. Otherwise, irreversible myocardial injury occurs.*

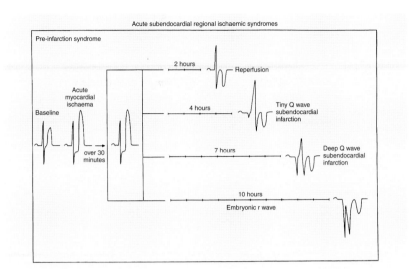

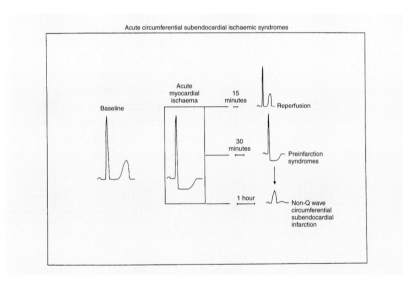

Figure 8.4 *The depth of the subendocardial infarction depends on the duration of obstruction. The range of ECG manifestations extends from the tiny qRs syndrome to the QrS syndrome (embryonic R wave syndrome).*

Figure 8.5 *Circumferential subendocardial ischaemia. In this syndrome, the window of opportunity is very short, and in most cases the outcome is dire. Surviving patients develop non-Q wave circumferential subendocardial infarction.*

Non-Q wave acute myocardial infarction

CASE 1

Non-Q-wave anterior acute myocardial infarction with ST segment depression and negative T-waves

A 79-year-old woman suffering from hypertension, diabetes mellitus and obesity who underwent coronary artery bypass surgery 4 years before the present admission. During the month before hospitalization she suffered from progressive angina, which evolved to rest angina and dyspnea during the week before admission. The first ECG was obtained on 22 July 1997 at 01.00, one hour after resolution of chest pain (*Fig. 8.6*). The ECG shows signs of left ventricular hypertrophy, with ST segment depression in the precordial leads V2–V6 and negative T waves. The P wave in lead V1 suggests enlargement of the left atrium.

The second ECG was obtained half an hour later (*Fig. 8.7*), without the patient having recurrence of pain and shows new inversion of the T-waves in leads I and aVL and the negative T waves in leads V2–V6 became deeper than in the first ECG.

A third ECG, obtained 7 hours later (*Fig. 8.8*), shows deepening of the T waves in the precordial leads.

The serum creatine kinase level was 220 IU on admission and 58 IU on the second day.

The two-dimensional echocardiogram obtained on 23 July 1997 (8 hours after admission) (*Fig. 8.9*) revealed normal-sized left ventricle. No regional wall motion abnormalities were detected. There is left atrial enlargement. The ECG (*Fig. 8.10*) was recorded during a severe angina pain at the coronary care unit. Note that the ST segment is becoming deeper maximally in V4 and V5 (4 mm). This is the typical pattern of circumferential subendocardial ischaemia.

A coronary angiography was performed immediately. This showed severe triple vessel coronary artery disease and a 99% diameter stenosis in a vein graft supplying the first obtuse marginal branch of the left circumflex artery. The left internal mammary artery, supplying the distal part of the left anterior descending coronary artery, was patent.

Comments
This patient shows a typical pattern of non-Q wave myocardial infarction, revealed by prolonged pain, mild increase and decrease in serum creatine kinase levels, and serial ST–T changes in leads LI, aVL, and the precordial leads. The ST segment depression in leads LI, aVL and V2–V6, indicates that this patient has diffuse coronary artery disease with elevated left ventricular end-diastolic pressure. The re-ischaemia usually developed by these patients is the circumferential subendocardial type, indicating a sudden increase in the diastolic pressure in the left ventricle induced by severe triple vessel disease or left main coronary artery disease. Urgent coronary angiography is highly recommended.

Percutaneous transluminal coronary angioplasty was performed to the thrombotic stenosis on the venous graft bypassed to the marginal one of the left circumflex artery.

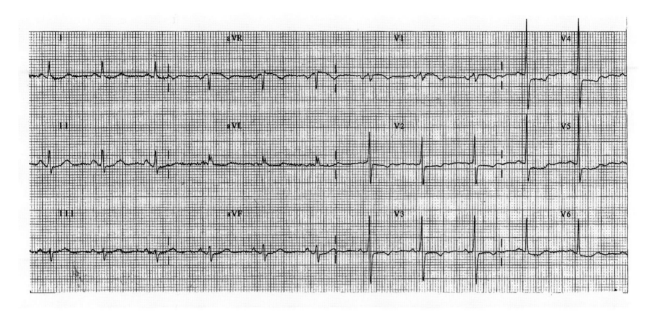

Figure 8.6 *ECG showing ST segment depression with inverted T waves with maximal ST-T changes in leads V4–V5, suggesting preinfarction syndrome of circumferential subendocardial ischaemia.*

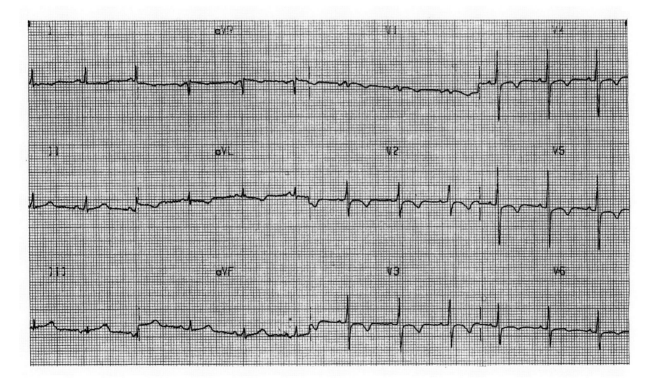

Figure 8.7 *ECG showing signs of complete reperfusion, inverted T waves in leads V2–V5 with 1 mm ST segment depression.*

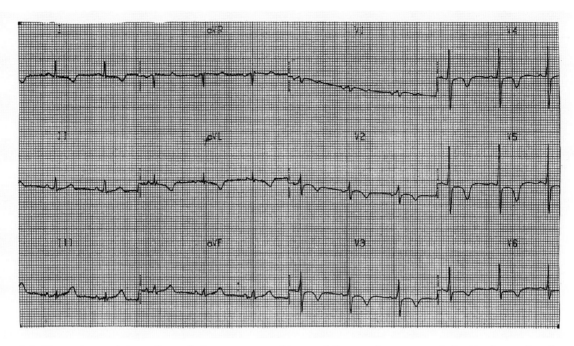

Figure 8.8 *More advanced signs of reperfusion; pronounced inverted T waves (non q wave infarction); reperfused non Q infarction with ST segment depression in leads V3–V6.*

DIAGNOSIS:
CORONARY ARTERY DISEASE
98% STENOSIS OF LEFT MAIN CORONARY ARTERY
100% STENOSIS OF LEFT ANTERIOR DECENDING ARTERY-PROXIMAL
100% STENOSIS OF LEFT CIRCUMFLEX ARTERY-PROXIMAL
100% STENOSIS OF RIGHT CORONARY ARTERY-PROXIMAL
99% STENOSIS OF VENOUS GRAFT TO CXMARGI

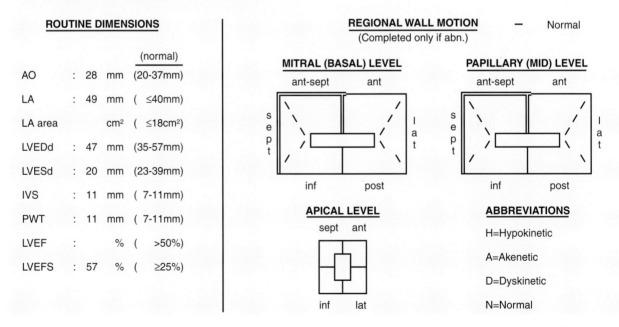

ROUTINE DIMENSIONS

				(normal)
AO	:	28	mm	(20-37mm)
LA	:	49	mm	(≤40mm)
LA area			cm²	(≤18cm²)
LVEDd	:	47	mm	(35-57mm)
LVESd	:	20	mm	(23-39mm)
IVS	:	11	mm	(7-11mm)
PWT	:	11	mm	(7-11mm)
LVEF	:		%	(>50%)
LVEFS	:	57	%	(≥25%)

REGIONAL WALL MOTION — Normal
(Completed only if abn.)

MITRAL (BASAL) LEVEL
ant-sept   ant
sept   lat
inf   post

PAPILLARY (MID) LEVEL
ant-sept   ant
sept   lat
inf   post

APICAL LEVEL
sept ant
inf   lat

ABBREVIATIONS

H=Hypokinetic

A=Akenetic

D=Dyskinetic

N=Normal

Figure 8.9 *A schematic presentation of the two-dimensional transthoracic echocardiographic examination performed 8 hours after admission. On the right side, the regional wall motion is divided schematically into 16 segments according to the conventions of the American Society of Echocardiography. No regional wall motion abnormality was recorded. On the left side, left heart dimensions, measured in M-mode long parasternal view, are depicted. There is left atrial enlargement (49 mm), whereas left ventricular size in systole and diastole are normal.*

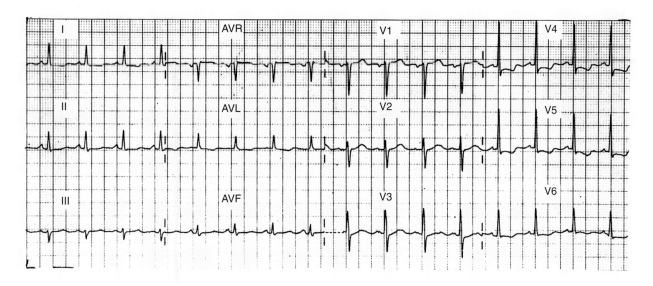

Figure 8.10 *ECG showing circumferential subendocardial ischaemia pattern during re-ischaemia*

CASE 2

Non-Q wave anterior acute myocardial infarction evolving to subendocardial regional myocardial infarction

A 49-year-old man suffering from stable angina on effort in the past year was admitted on 18 July 1992 to the cardiac intensive care unit 4 hours after the onset of chest pain. The first ECG was obtained at 06.00 (*Fig. 8.11*).

PREINFARCTION STRATIFICATION

The ECG showed preinfarction syndrome (no Q waves), with transmural ischaemia (ST-segment elevation), regional ischaemia (tall T waves), and anterior wall ischaemia (visible in the precordial leads).

CORONARY ANATOMY

- The culprit artery is the left anterior descending coronary artery (LAD), (maximal ischaemic changes in leads V2–V3).
- The level of obstruction is distal to the first diagonal artery (D1) (isoelectric ST-segment T wave.
- The dimensions of the LAD are type B: (lead LIII shows isoelectric ST segment.

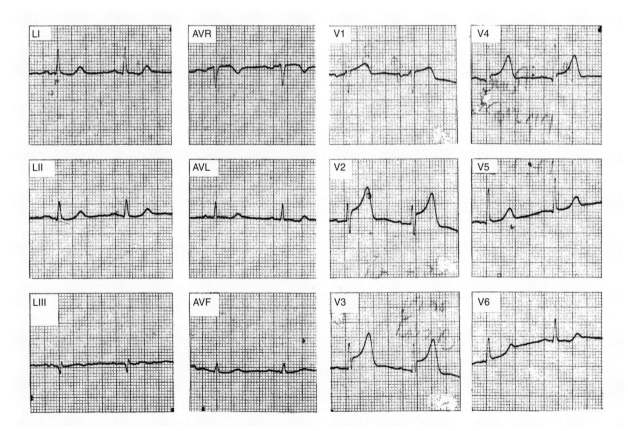

Figure 8.11 *ECG showing preinfarction syndrome of transmural regional anterior wall.*

MYOCARDIAL ANATOMY

- The core of the myocardial ischaemia is moderate (ST segment elevation in leads V2–V3 only).
- The border zone is large: there is Grade 1 ischaemia in leads V4–V6 (probably because of overlapping circulation from the obtuse marginal branches of the left circumflex artery).
- The right side of the septum is involved (in lead V1, there are ST segment elevation and positive T waves; this area is most probably supplied by the LAD).

PHYSIOLOGY

Grade 2 ischaemia is shown in leads V2 and V3 (indicating moderate protection). Grade 1 ischaemia is shown in V4–V6 (indicating well protected areas).

The patient received heparin and aspirin and was admitted to the cardiac intensive care unit. A second ECG was performed 2 hours later at 08.00 (*Fig. 8.12*). It showed non-Q wave myocardial infarction. The ST segments are isoelectric and the T waves are inverted in the precordial leads.

On 19 July 1992 at 08.00, a similar pattern was noted (*Fig. 8.13*). Two hours later, the patient experienced severe pain, and a pseudonormalization of the T waves was noted (*Fig. 8.14*). After intravenous administration of nitrates, signs of reperfusion were seen (a decrease in the magnitude of the T waves) (*Fig. 8.15*). Two hours later (*Fig. 8.16*), the T waves became negative.

The following day (20 July 1992) at 08.00, the ECG showed newly developed Q waves (*Fig. 8.17*). qrs complexes are seen in leads V2 and V3. There is no diminution of the R waves in these leads. This is a sign of regional subendocardial infarction (see Chapter 4).

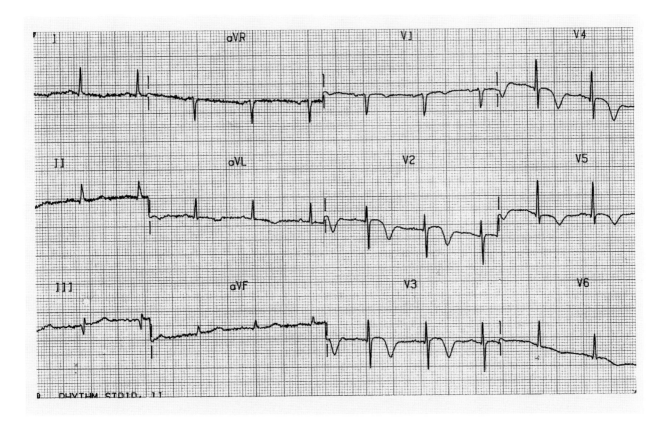

Figure 8.12 *ECG showing complete reperfusion signs; inverted T waves with isoelectric ST segments in the involved leads.*

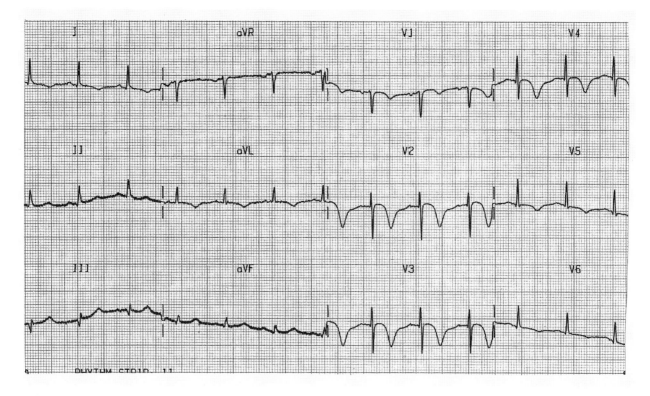

Figure 8.13 *Pattern of reperfusion; non Q wave infarction with isoelectric ST segment.*

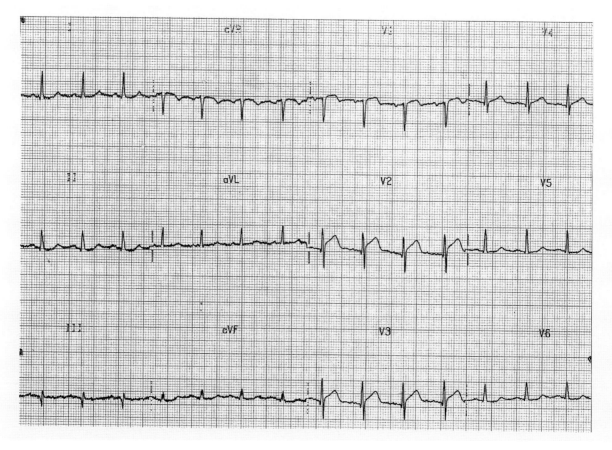

Figure 8.14 *Transmural regional re-ischaemia; re-elevation of ST segment in leads V2–V3 with positivation of the T waves, V4–V5–V6 'pseudonormalization'.*

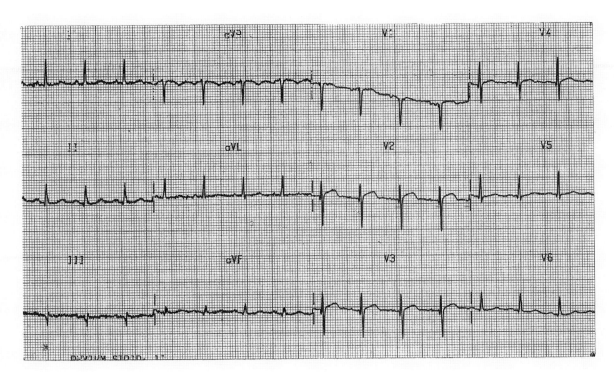

Figure 8.15 *ECG showing first stage of reperfusion; the ST-T waves decrease in their magnitude in leads V2–V3 as well as in leads V4–V6. Tiny T waves appear in leads V2–V3–V4 indicating a more advanced grade of infaction – regional subendocardial infarction.*

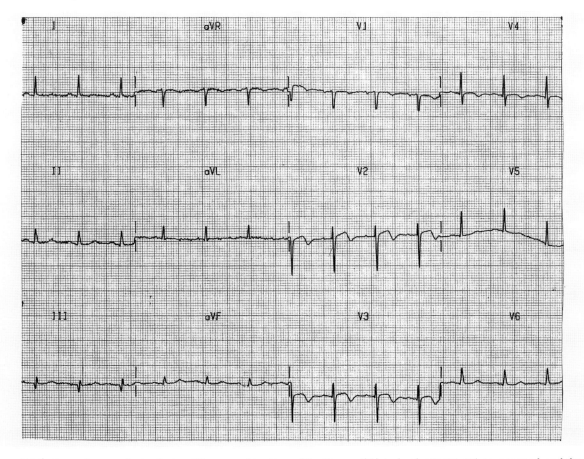

Figure 8.16 *Second stage of reperfusion. The second portion of the T wave (T_2) in leads V2–V3–V4 are inverted and the first portion (T_1) and the ST segment are elevated 1–2 mm.*

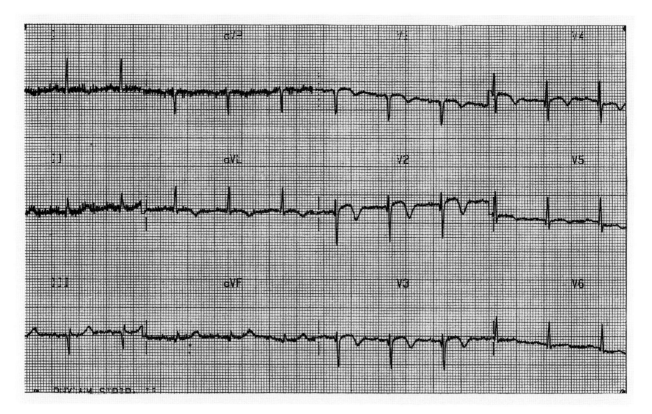

Figure 8.17 *Third stage of reperfusion. Negative T waves with isoelectric ST segment in leads V3–V6–V2 with 1 mm elevation.*

Coronary angiography (on 21 July 1992) showed 95% diameter stenosis with angiographic evidence of a thrombus in the left anterior descending coronary artery distal to the origin of the first diagonal branch (*Fig. 8.18*). TIMI grade 3 flow was noted. The left anterior descending coronary artery reaches the apex but does not wrap it (type B). There is no right conal branch (*Fig. 8.19*).

Comments

This case shows two types of infarctions in a well-protected myocardium. Despite being recorded after 4 hours of chest pain, the first ECG (preinfarction) shows only Grade 2 ischaemia in leads V2 and V3 and Grade 1 ischaemia in leads V4–V6. The patient experienced reperfusion after administration of heparin and aspirin. According to the ECG (see *Figs 8.12 and 8.13*) the patient had complete reperfusion (negative deep T waves with isoelectric ST segments in all the leads that showed Grade 1 or Grade 2 ischaemia on the initial ECG), and no Q waves evolved.

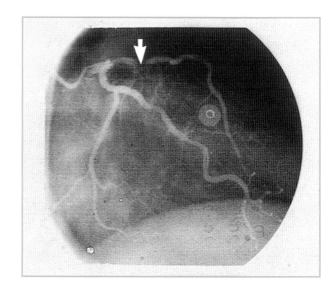

Figure 8.18 *Right anterior oblique view of the left coronary system. Arrow shows the critical obstruction of the LAD with reperfusion TIMI 3. The large marginal artery overlaps the anterolateral wall.*

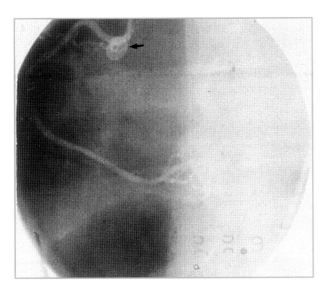

Figure 8.19 *Left anterior oblique view of the right coronary artery; no conal artery is seen.*

The ECG obtained during recurrence of pain (see *Fig. 8.14*) shows that the infarct-related artery was re-occluded: there was re-elevation of the ST segment and pseudo-positivation of the T waves in leads V2 and V3 (Grade 2 ischaemia) and positivation of the T waves, without ST segment elevation in lead V1 or leads V4–V6 (Grade 1 ischaemia). After resolution of pain, progressive changes were observed in the T waves, which became negative (see *Figs 8.15 and 8.16*), whereas only minor changes were seen in the amplitude of the ST segment elevation. This time, reperfusion was incomplete, since there was no complete resolution of the ST segment elevation. Despite similar ischaemic time (4 hours) to the first episode, new q waves appeared this time, probably due to incomplete reperfusion. These q waves are a sign of subendocardial infarction and differ from the q waves of transmural infarction (qS waves) (see Chapter 4).

This case demonstrates the need for repeating the ECG recording whenever there is a change in the clinical situation. Evaluation and risk stratification should be performed each time an ECG is obtained.

In this type of regional transmural re-ischaemia there is no need for an emergency invasive procedure as there was in the first case described.

CASE 3

Non-Q wave acute myocardial infarction without adequate reperfusion

A 68-year-old man with hypertension was admitted because of unstable angina with prolonged chest pain. The first ECG was obtained on 26 January 1997 at 22.00 (*Fig. 8.20*). In this recording, the acute myocardial ischaemic changes were subtle and easy to misdiagnose. The ST segment elevation in lead V1 with positive T waves is frequently seen in patients with chronic hypertension, as is the ST segment depression in leads V5 and V6.

The patient's chest pain resolved and did not recur. The next ECG was obtained on 27 January 1997 at 08.00 (*Fig. 8.21*) and showed ST segment elevation with positive T1 waves (the first part of the T wave; see Chapters 2 and 3) and negative T2 waves (the second part of the T wave) in leads V2–V4. ST segment elevation with negative T waves was seen in leads V4 and V5.

The following day, further changes in the precordial leads were seen (*Fig. 8.22*). The negative T waves

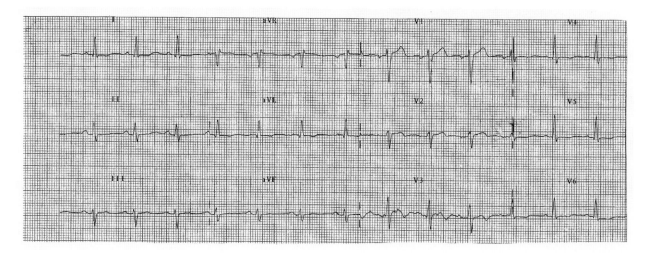

Figure 8.20 *ECG recorded during prolonged anginal pain. No diagnosis of ST–T changes for acute ischaemic heart disease.*

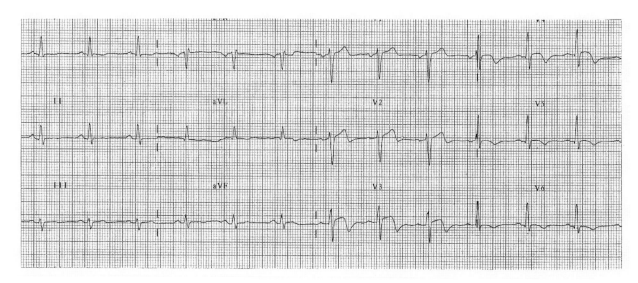

Figure 8.21 *ECG showing 2nd stage of reperfusion making evident the ischaemia in leads V2–V6; inverted T₂; ST segment and T₁ waves elevation.*

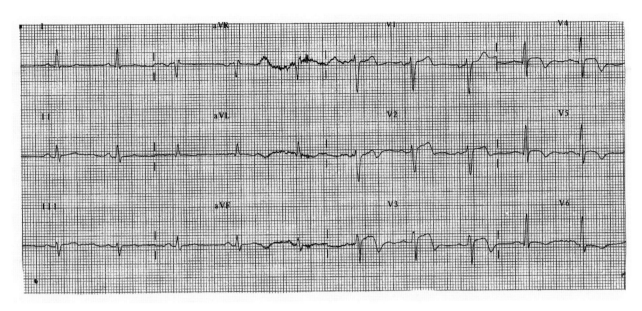

Figure 8.22 *ECG showing non-Q-wave infarction of anterior wall with incomplete reperfusion.*

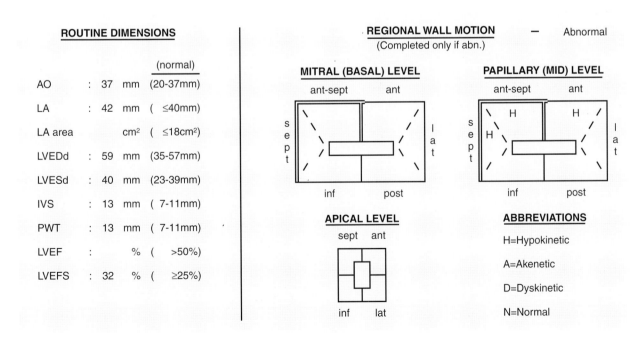

ROUTINE DIMENSIONS			
			(normal)
AO	:	37 mm	(20-37mm)
LA	:	42 mm	(≤40mm)
LA area		cm²	(≤18cm²)
LVEDd	:	59 mm	(35-57mm)
LVESd	:	40 mm	(23-39mm)
IVS	:	13 mm	(7-11mm)
PWT	:	13 mm	(7-11mm)
LVEF	:	%	(>50%)
LVEFS	:	32 %	(≥25%)

REGIONAL WALL MOTION   —   Abnormal
(Completed only if abn.)

MITRAL (BASAL) LEVEL

PAPILLARY (MID) LEVEL

APICAL LEVEL

ABBREVIATIONS

H=Hypokinetic

A=Akenetic

D=Dyskinetic

N=Normal

Figure 8.23 *ECG showing hypokinesia of the low anteroseptal and anterior wall.*

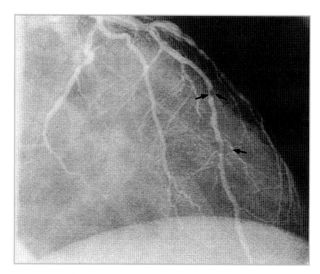

Figure 8.24 *Coronary angiography: right anterior oblique view of the left system showing the level of obstruction of the left anterior descending artery, the first proximal and the second very distal.*

became deeper. This pattern was recorded during the next 3 days. After 4 days, the patient developed chest pain. ECG recordings obtained during pain showed positivation of the T waves in the precordial leads.

Serum creatine kinase was elevated, and two-dimensional echocardiography (*Fig. 8.23*) showed akinesis in the apical septum and anterior segments

and hypokinesis of the mid-anterior and anteroseptal segments.

Coronary angiography (*Fig. 8.24*) shows several narrowing lesions in the left anterior descending coronary artery (see the coronary angiography report). The two levels of left anterior descending artery obstruction are emphasized by two black arrows (*Fig. 8.24*).

Comments

This case shows another type of non-Q wave myocardial infarction. In contrast to the previous cases, in which resolution of the ST segment elevation with negative T waves was observed, in this case the pattern of persistence of the ST segment elevation and negative T waves indicates incomplete reperfusion, probably because of serial narrowings of the left anterior descending coronary artery.

In this case the coronary anatomy cannot be determined by the ECG because there was no ECG in the preinfarction syndrome stage. If there is no ECG in the acute preinfarction syndrome stage, the exact site of the culprit lesion, the size of the infarct related artery, and the size and location of the myocardial ischaemic area at risk cannot be appreciated.

This type of non-Q wave infarction is prone to develop re-ischaemia; some cases are difficult to solve because the distal obstruction is almost in the terminal portion of the left anterior descending artery.

CASE 4

The malignant non-Q wave acute myocardial infarction

A 60-year-old man with hypertensive heart disease and stable angina for many years was admitted to an internal medicine ward because of unstable angina. The first ECG was obtained on 11 December 1996 (*Fig. 8.25*). This ECG is of poor quality, but it shows non-specific T wave changes in leads LI, aVL and V4–V6. There is poor progression of the R waves in leads V1–V3.

Two hours later the patient developed chest pain and shortness of breath. The ECG obtained at this time (*Fig. 8.26*) shows ST segment depression in leads LI, aVL, and V5 and V6, with negative T waves.

The patient was transferred to the cardiac intensive care unit. On arrival, he was in severe respiratory distress with pulmonary oedema. The ECG obtained at this time shows complete left bundle branch block (*Fig. 8.27*).

The patient was intubated and mechanically venti-lated and an intra-aortic balloon pump was intro-duced. The patient was taken immediately to the catheterization laboratory. Coronary angiography showed 98% left main coronary artery stenosis, severe stenosis (85%) of the proximal left anterior descending coronary artery, and 90% stenosis of the proximal left circumflex artery (*Fig. 8.28*). The patient underwent emergency coronary artery bypass surgery. Immediately after surgery, the ECG showed non-Q wave myocardial infarction with incomplete left bundle branch block pattern (*Fig. 8.29*).

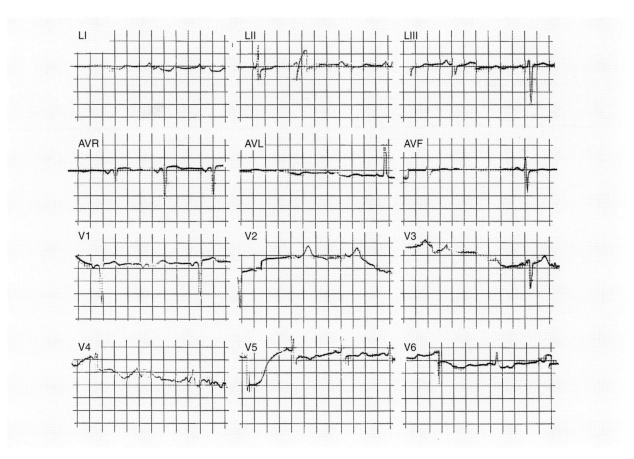

Figure 8.25 *ECG showing unspecific ST–T changes in leads V4–V5 and a poor progression of the r wave in leads V2–V4.*

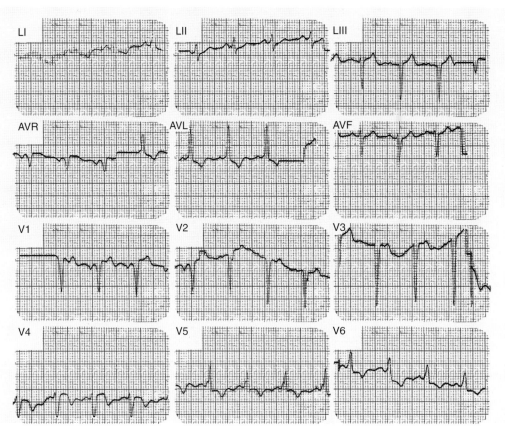

Figure 8.26 *ECG recorded during pain and severe respiratory distress showing circumferential subendocardial preinfarction syndrome.*

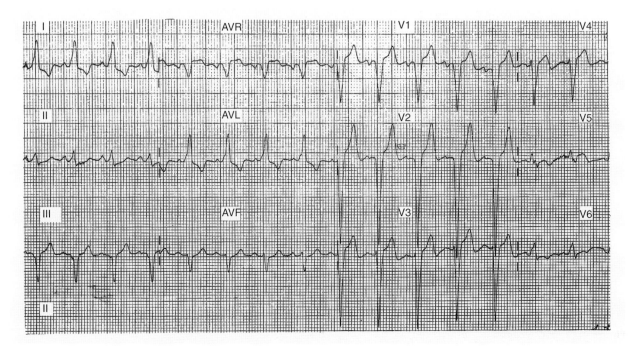

Figure 8.27 *Complete LBBB during severe pulmonary oedema (traction block).*

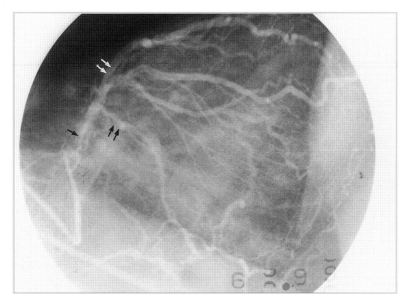

Figure 8.28 *Coronary angiography showing severe left main (single arrow) and left main (double arrows) equivalent obstruction.*

Comments

This is a typical ECG pattern of a circumferential non-Q wave myocardial infarction, for there is ST segment depression with negative T waves in leads V4–V6 without ST segment elevation in other leads (as was extensively discussed in Chapter 4). This pattern represents an ominous course and mandates immediate evaluation and intervention. The site of the culprit lesion cannot be evaluated; however, this pattern represents either left main coronary artery infarction or infarction in a patient with critically narrowed proximal left anterior descending and left circumflex coronary arteries (left main equivalent syndrome).

In this case the appearance of new left bundle branch block indicates extreme dilatation of the left ventricle (i.e. traction block; see Chapter 7).

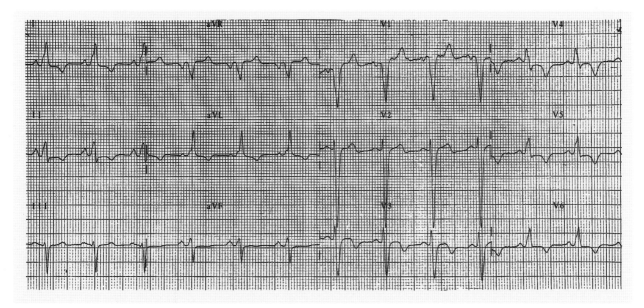

Figure 8.29 *ECG recorded a few hours after CABG; non-Q-wave infarction, circumferential subendocardial infarction. Note the wide QRS complex; reappearance of r waves in leads V2–V4 and ST segment depression with inverted T waves in leads V4–V6.*

CASE 5

Acute myocardial infarction with Grade 1 ischaemia (no ST segment elevation)

A 70-year-old man with hypercholesterolaemia, an inferior wall acute myocardial infarction 5 years before the present admission, and chronic stable angina was admitted after 6 hours of precordial pain on 16 December 1996. The first ECG was recorded at 17.00 (*Fig. 8.30*).

PREINFARCTION STRATIFICATION

The ECG showed preinfarction syndrome (no Q waves) with regional ischaemia (positive, tall and peaked T waves) and anterior wall ischaemia (shown in the precordial leads).

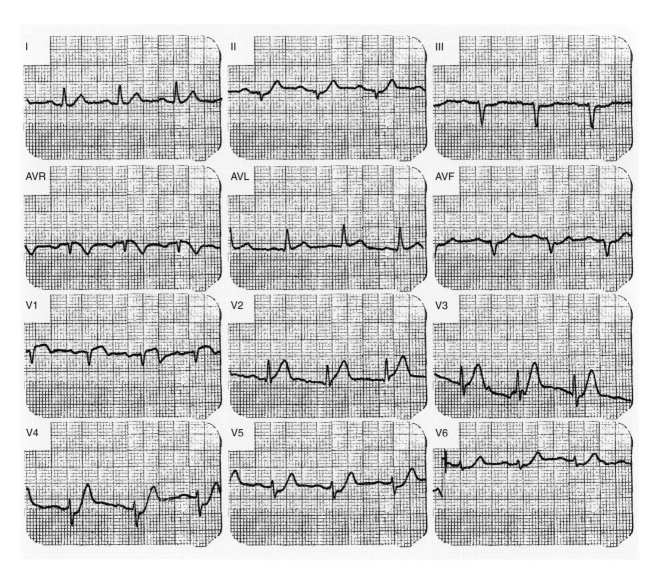

Figure 8.30 *Preinfarction syndrome, transmural regional in leads V2–V3 (non-Q-waves, ST segment elevation, positive T waves); in leads V4–V5 subendocardial regional (ST segment depression and positive T waves). Extreme left axis deviation in the frontal plane.*

CORONARY ANATOMY

- The culprit artery is the left anterior descending artery (LAD) (maximal changes in leads V2 and V3).
- The level of obstruction is proximal to the D1 (moderate ST segment elevation and positive T waves in lead aVL).
- The dimension of the artery is type C (moderate ST segment depression with positive T waves; the T waves in lead aVL are smaller than in lead L1; there is an attenuation phenomenon between leads aVL and LIII) (see Chapter 2).

MYOCARDIAL ANATOMY

- The core of infarction is small, seen in lead V2 only; leads V3–V6 show regional subendocardial ischaemia (ST segment depression with tall and peaked T-waves).
- This border zone shows a highly protected area, in which only the subendocardial area is affected (maximal protection in the subepicardial area).

- The right side of the septum is not involved (lead V1 shows reciprocal changes to the subendocardial ischaemia of lead V6—i.e. ST segment elevation with negative T waves).

PHYSIOLOGY

- Grade 1 ischaemia in lead V2 and Grade 2 subendocardial regional ischaemia in leads V3–V6 (see Chapter 1). This represents maximally protected myocardium, probably because of well developed collateral vessels.

Twelve hours later (*Fig. 8.31*), signs of reperfusion appeared. The T waves in lead V2 became less positive and the ST segment in the precordial leads became isoelectric while the T waves decreased in amplitude (but remained positive).

An additional ECG obtained 13 hours later (*Fig. 8.32*) shows that these changes progressed. The changes in the precordial R wave amplitudes are due to different positioning of the leads in a patient with

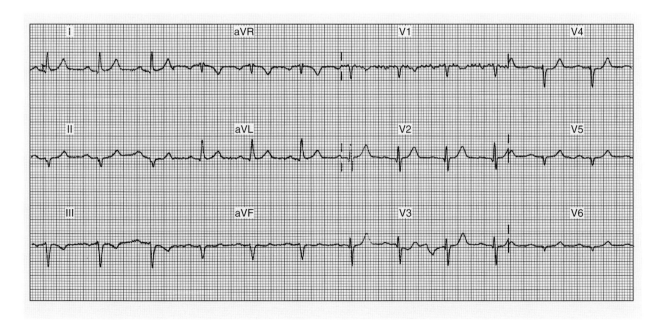

Figure 8.31 *First stage of reperfusion; isoelectric ST segments in leads V3–V6 with decrease in the magnitude of the T waves.*

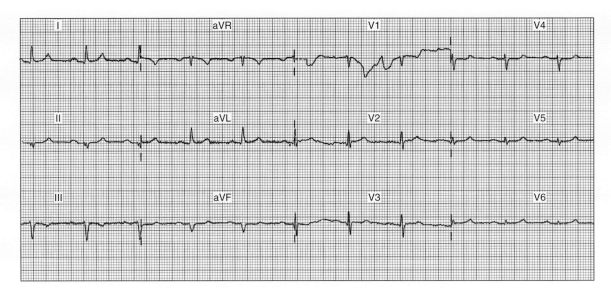

Figure 8.32 *Further decrease in the magnitude of the T waves in the precordial leads.*

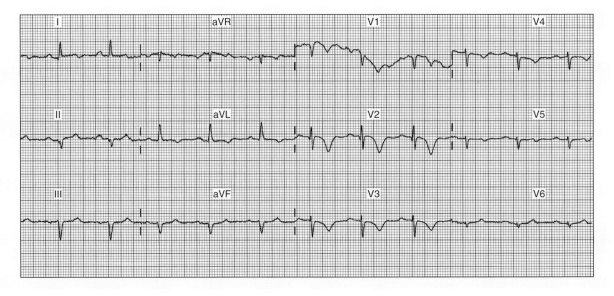

Figure 8.33 *Subendocardial regional infarction (tiny q waves in leads V2–V3) with complete reperfusion (inverted T waves in the precordial leads).*

left axis deviation (see Chapter 5); however, no Q waves developed (*Fig. 8.33*).

After an additional 12 hours (*Fig. 8.34*), there was inversion of the T waves in leads LI, aVL, and V1–V5 and development of new Q waves in leads V2–V3.

Two-dimensional echocardiography performed on 18 December 1996, revealed akinesis of the mid- and apical anteroseptal and anterior segments of the left ventricle (*Fig. 8.35*). Coronary angiography obtained on 20 December 1996 (*Fig. 8.36*) showed proximal occlusion of the left anterior descending coronary artery and a large obtuse marginal branch supplied by collateral vessels from the distal part of the left anterior descending artery (*Fig. 8.36b*). This marginal branch protected the distal anterolateral segments (see Chapter 3). The right coronary (*Fig. 8.36a*) gives two branches that supply the right septum with a large conal branch. After balloon angioplasty was performed (*Fig. 8.37*), the left anterior descending artery is shown to be a long artery that wraps around the apex (i.e. type C).

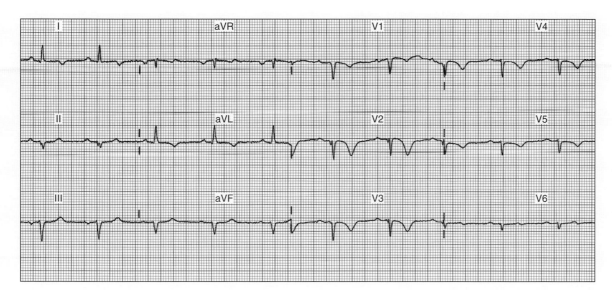

Figure 8.34 *Further decrease of the r wave in leads V2–V3 with tiny q waves; complete reperfusion (inverted T waves and isoelectric ST segments.*

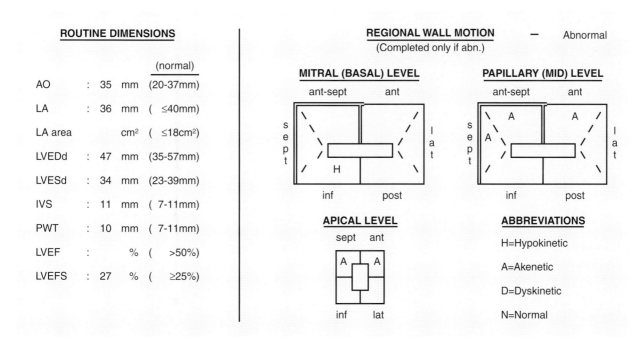

Figure 8.35 *Echocardiogram showing akinesia in the apical, mid-anteroseptal and anterior wall.*

Comments

This is an ECG of a preinfarction syndrome showing a myocardium that is highly protected by its collateral circulation. Despite having sudden proximal left anterior descending coronary artery obstruction, there is Grade 1 ischaemia only in lead V2, whereas in leads V3–V6 there is subendocardial ischaemia. Collateral circulation from the big obtuse marginal branch probably prevented transmural ischaemia. In this case, signs of reperfusion developed relatively late, because reperfusion occurred by recruitment of collateral vessels and not by recanalization of the

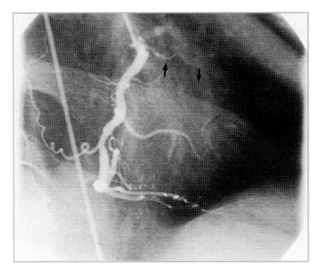

a

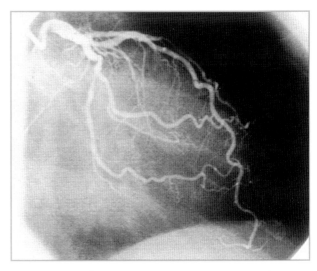

Figure 8.37 *After angioplasty, a LAD-type C is evident.*

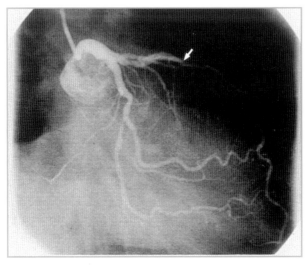

b

Figure 8.36 *(a) Coronary angiography: right anterior oblique view showing a conal artery that supplies the right septum. (b) Total obstruction of the LAD. Note the big marginal artery supplying the anterolateral wall and the collateral supplying the third portion of the LAD.*

culprit lesion. This case represents an interesting finding in that Q waves can evolve even in patients without ST segment elevation in the acute stage, as was discussed in Chapter 3. In addition, Q waves may evolve relatively late; therefore classification into Q wave or non-Q wave myocardial infarction cannot be made during the first 48–72 hours.

CASE 6

Mid-ventricular non-Q wave myocardial infarction

A 56-year-old woman without a prior history of heart disease presented on 29 January 1996 at 10.30 with severe angina that had persisted for 90 minutes. The first ECG (*Fig. 8.38*) depicts preinfarction syndrome (non-Q wave), transmural regional ischaemia (tall and peaked T waves), and anterior wall ischaemia (seen in leads V2, LI, and aVL).

PREINFARCTION STRATIFICATION

CORONARY ANATOMY

Maximal changes in leads LI and aVL with ST segment depression and inverted T waves in lead LIII suggest that the artery supplying the mid-ventricle is narrowed. This artery may be a diagonal branch, a marginal branch, or an intermediate branch. The elevation in lead V2 only in the precordial leads suggests that the diagonal branch is the culprit. It is possible that the left anterior descending

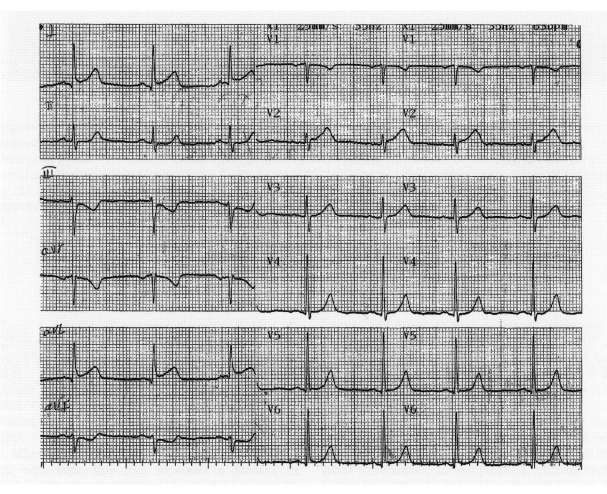

Figure 8.38 *Preinfarction syndrome, transmural regional of the mid-anterior wall. ST segment elevation in leads LI, a VL and V2 with positive T waves; ST segment depression in leads LIII and VF with negative T waves (reciprocal changes).*

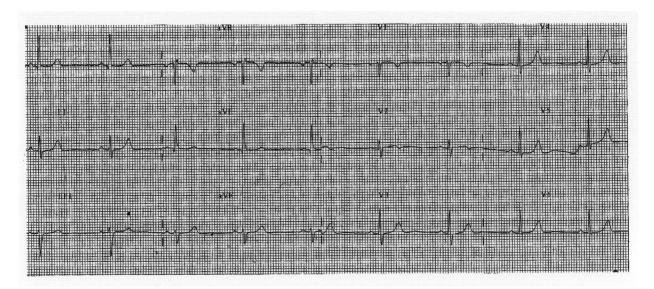

Figure 8.39 *First stage of reperfusion; isoelectric ST segment in the involved leads with a decrease in the T waves.*

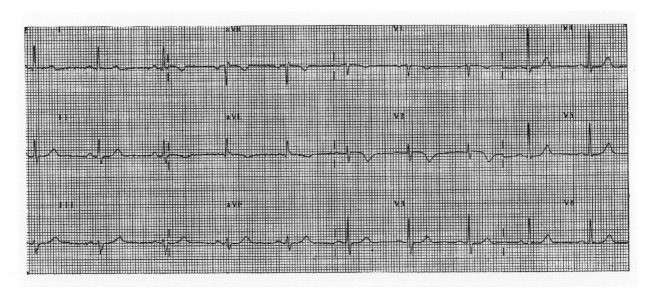

Figure 8.40 *Complete non-Q-wave infarction of the mid-anterior wall with complete reperfusion (inverted T waves in lead V2). Note the decrease in the magnitude of the R waves in leads LI and aVL.*

coronary artery is also involved, although there are no ECG signs of this. The tall, peaked T waves in leads V3–V6 with slight ST segment depression suggest that the obstruction is restricted to the diagonal branch. The dimensions of the artery and the level of the obstruction cannot be determined because the culprit artery is a secondary epicardial vessel and not a major vessel.

The patient received intravenous heparin and oral aspirin. Thrombolytic therapy was not given. There were signs of reperfusion in the second ECG (*Fig. 8.39*), which was obtained 90 minutes after the first ECG. There was resolution of the ST segment elevation in leads LI, aVL, and V2 and resolution of ST segment depression in lead LIII. The T wave in the precordial leads and the involved leads decreased in amplitude.

The third ECG was obtained at 14.00 on the same day (*Fig. 8.40*). More advanced stages of reperfusion are evident with inverted T waves in lead aVL and deep, inverted T waves in lead V2. This is the last stage of reperfusion.

Echocardiography performed the following day did not detect any abnormality in regional wall motion. Coronary angiography performed 2 days after the acute episode revealed a severe narrowing in a small diagonal branch.

Comments

This is a typical example of mid-ventricular infarction caused by a spontaneous, isolated obstruction. This may also occur during angioplasty when a side branch is compromised. To recognize this type of infarction sestamibi scintigraphy should be performed (see Chapter 2).

CASE 7

Inferior wall and the S1Q3 syndrome

A 42-year-old man was admitted to the coronary care unit on 2 March 1997 with a 2-hour history of severe chest pain. The patient received analgesics, intravenous heparin, and nitroglycerine. The pain resolved. The ECG obtained upon admission at 05.00 (*Fig. 8.41*) shows an S1Q3 pattern in inferior leads and moderate ST segment elevation of 1 mm in leads LII, LIII, and aVF. Slight ST segment depression was appreciated in lead aVL with an isoelectric T wave. This pattern is highly suspicious of inferior wall infarction.

Two hours later (*Fig. 8.42*), the T wave in lead LIII was inverted and isoelectric in lead aVF. In lead aVL, the T wave became more positive and the ST segment became isoelectric. The next day an inverted T wave in lead III was seen. No changes were seen in other leads (*Fig. 8.43*).

The creatine kinase upon admission was 700 U. On the third day the creatine kinase returned to normal.

An echocardiogram revealed hypokinesia in the inferior wall without any abnormality in the dimensions of the heart nor any valvular disease (*Fig. 8.44*). Coronary angiography revealed a 90% distal narrowing of a small right coronary artery.

Comments

This type of diagnostic challenge is common and is discussed in Chapter 2. Despite the presence of the Q wave in lead LIII, this type of infarction should be regarded as non-Q wave; in other words, the Q wave is not pathological but rather reflects the orientation of the heart in the chest.

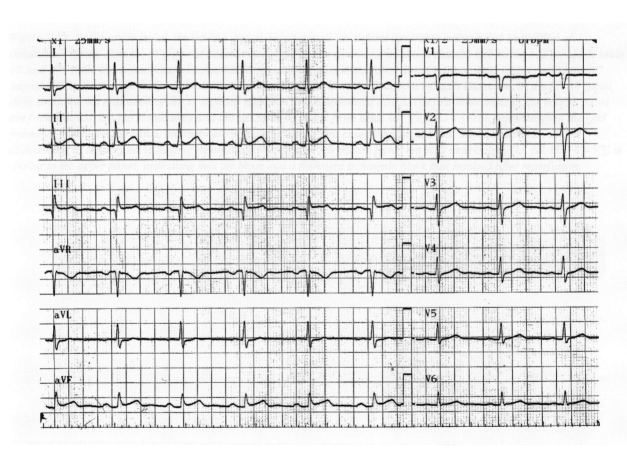

Figure 8.41 *Preinfarction syndrome of the inferior wall in the presence of S1-q3 pattern. Note, ST segment elevation in lead LIII (1 mm) and positive T waves.*

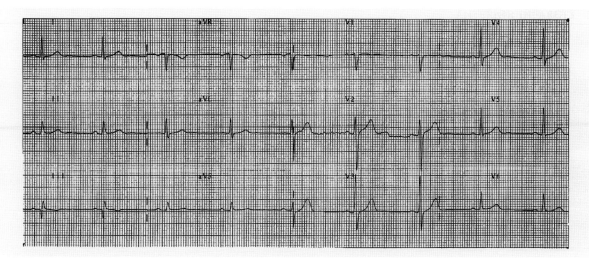

Figure 8.42 *First stage of reperfusion: isoelectric ST segment with isoelectric T wave in lead LIII.*

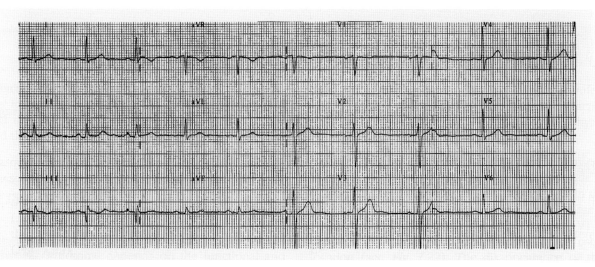

Figure 8.43 *Non-Q-wave infarction with incomplete reperfusion. Note the decrease of the r wave in lead aVF. The R wave in LIII is positional.*

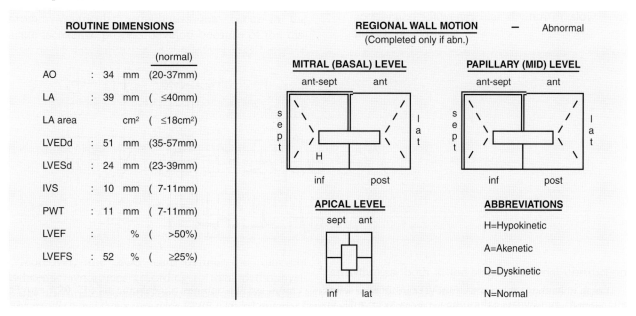

Figure 8.44 *ECG showing hypokinesia in a very small area of the inferior wall.*

CASE 8

Non-Q wave infarction and extreme left axis deviation

A 78-year-old man with prior inferior wall infarction was hospitalized with progressive rest angina. On 15 July 1997 he awoke with severe chest pain, which lasted 2 hours. The first ECG was obtained at 07.30 and showed anterior regional preinfarction syndrome (*Fig. 8.45*).

PREINFARCTION STRATIFICATION

The ECG showed preinfarction syndrome with no Q waves (the small r waves in leads V2 and V3 are an expression of the extreme left axis deviation in the frontal plane; this depends on the location of the right precordial leads), transmural ischaemia (ST segment elevation), and regional ischaemia (tall and peaked T waves).

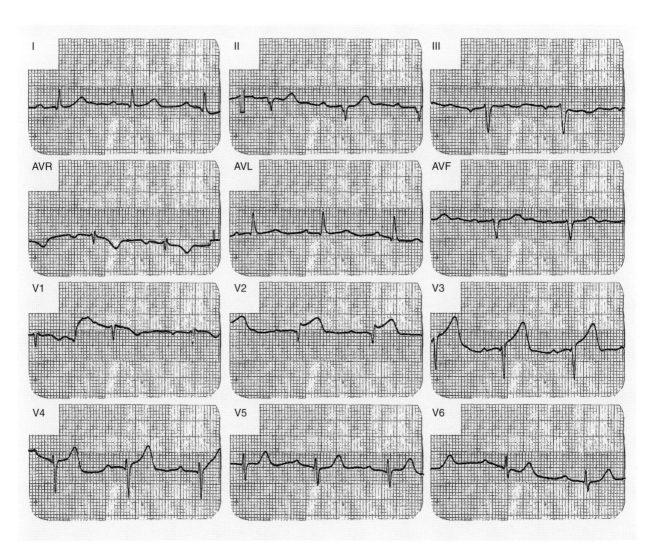

Figure 8.45 *ECG showing an extreme left axis deviation with inferior wall infarction (no r wave in lead LII). The precordial leads show preinfarction syndrome with ST segment elevation in leads V2–V3 and positive T waves. There is correlation between the Q wave in lead V2 and the ischaemia of the LAHB.*

CORONARY ANATOMY

- The culprit artery is the left anterior descending artery (LAD) (maximal changes in leads V2 and V3).
- The level of obstruction is distal to the first diagonal artery (D1) (no ST segment elevation in lead aVL).
- The dimension of the left anterior descending artery is probably type C (no shift in ST segment and T wave) in lead LIII. It is difficult to reach a correct evaluation because of the influence of the extreme left anterior hemiblock in the ST segment and the T waves in the standard leads.

MYOCARDIAL ANATOMY

- The core of the myocardial ischaemia is moderate (ST-segment elevation in leads V2 and V3).
- The border zone is large in leads V4–V6 (most probably because of overlapping circulation in the anterolateral wall by the second marginal artery of the circumflex artery).
- The right septum is not involved (isoelectric ST segment with negative T waves in lead V1; this area is probably supplied by the conal branch of the right coronary artery).

CORONARY PHYSIOLOGY

The myocardium is moderately protected, as suggested by the ischaemia Grade 2 type A pattern (see Chapter 2). Leads V5 and V6 show ST segment depression with positive T waves, suggesting that the subendocardial area is more involved than the subepicardial.

The patient received thrombolytic therapy. Two hours later, a second ECG was obtained (*Fig. 8.46*). There is evidence of re-ischaemia, with ST segment elevation in leads V2 and V3 (5 mm) and tall and peaked T waves (20 mm in lead V3). The T wave in leads V4–V6 also increased markedly in amplitude. Note the ST segment elevation in leads LI and aVL (though the amplitude of the T wave in LI is greater than in aVL). The dimension of the left anterior descending artery — type C is evident when the re-elevation of the ST segment and the T wave in lead LI is higher than ST segment and T wave in lead aVL (aVL attenuated by lead LIII). The ST segment re-elevation is consistent with reperfusion re-ischaemia (see Chapter 3).

After nitrates were given, a third ECG was obtained (*Fig. 8.47*). Signs of the initial stages of reperfusion were evident. In leads V2–V4 there is resolution of the ST segment elevation as well as of the tall T waves. Similar changes occurred in leads aVL and LI. The ST segment depression in leads V5 and V6 (subendocardial ischaemia) as well as in lead L3 (reciprocal change) resolved.

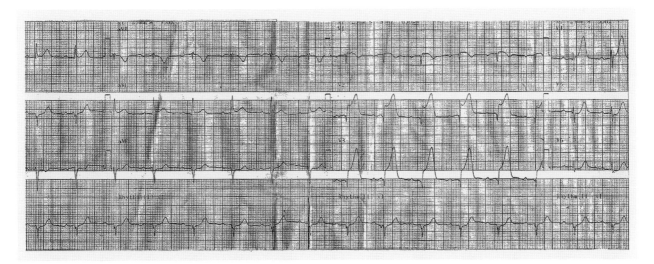

Figure 8.46 *Reperfusion re-ischaemia due to thrombolytic therapy. Note, re-elevation of the ST segment and the T waves in all the precordial leads (phasic flow variation).*

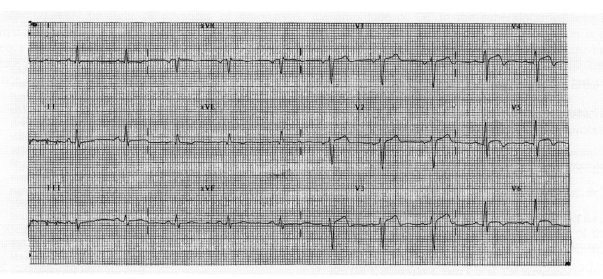

Figure 8.47 *First stage of reperfusion: ST segment elevation in leads V2–V4 with inverted T waves in leads V4–V5 and decrease in the magnitude of the T waves in leads V2–V3.*

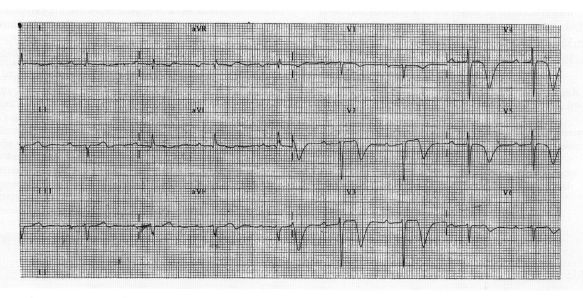

Figure 8.48 *Non-q-wave infarction with complete reperfusion; r waves in leads V3–V6; the r/s pattern in the precordial leads is a consequence of the extreme left anterior hemiblock (LAHB).*

The next day, a fourth ECG was obtained (*Fig. 8.48*). Signs of complete reperfusion were evident, as indicated by deep, inverted T waves and an isoelectric ST segment. The R wave in all precordial leads decreased in amplitude, which can partially be explained by the left axis deviation. The reduction in R wave amplitude indicates advanced stages of non-Q wave infarction.

Comments
The second ECG (see *Fig. 8.46*) is of particular significance. It depicts re-ischaemia caused by reperfusion.

The ST segment and T waves are of greater amplitude than they were before thrombolytic therapy. This re-ischaemia may be the result of the release of vasoactive agents, which cause cyclic flow variation. The small r wave in leads V2 and V3 can be explained by the shift of the vector to the left owing to the lateral wall ischaemia (see Chapter 2). The last tracing (see *Fig. 8.48*) depicts the persistent pattern of non-Q wave infarction in the precordial leads with an isoelectric ST-segment and inverted T waves.

CASE 9

QRS anterior wall subendocardial infarction

A 70-year-old woman was admitted to the coronary care unit after 4 hours of severe precordial pain. An ECG was obtained on 25 April 1997 at 02.00 (*Fig. 8.49*). Preinfarction syndrome was evident, with ST segment elevation (transmural and regional ischaemia) and tall and peaked T waves in the precordial leads.

PREINFARCTION STRATIFICATION

CORONARY ANATOMY

- The culprit artery is the left anterior descending artery (LAD) (maximal changes in leads V2 and V3).
- The level of obstruction is distal to the first diagonal artery (D1) (ST segment depression in lead aVL).
- The dimension of the artery is type C (wrapping around the apex), indicated by the ST segment elevation in lead LIII.

MYOCARDIAL ANATOMY

- The core of the myocardial ischaemia is moderate (ST segment elevation in leads V2 and V3).
- The border zone is large (tall T waves in leads V4–V6). The anterolateral wall is probably also supplied by a marginal branch.
- The right side of the septum is supplied by the left anterior descending coronary artery, indicated by the ST segment elevation and upright T waves in lead V1.

PHYSIOLOGY

The myocardium is moderately protected as evidenced by ischaemia Grade 2 type A (see Chapter 2). The anterolateral wall leads showed ischaemia Grade 1.

An ECG obtained 2 hours later (*Fig. 8.50*) manifests a unique type of reperfusion, namely resolution of the ST segment elevation with persistent upright T waves. A further ECG obtained 6 hours later (*Fig. 8.51*) showed an inverted T wave in the precordial leads (leads V1–V5) and lead LIII, and tiny q waves in leads V2 and V3. (This q wave represents subendocardial injury.)

An ECG obtained 2 days later (*Fig. 8.52*) showed

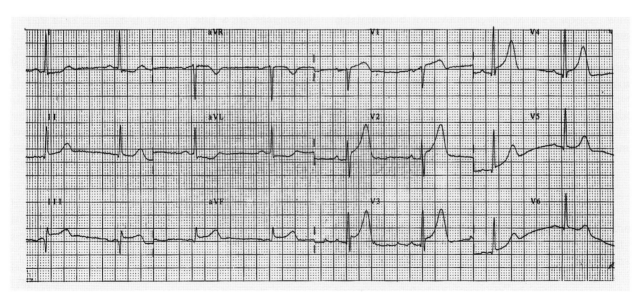

Figure 8.49 *ECG showing preinfarction syndrome, transmural regional anterior wall.*

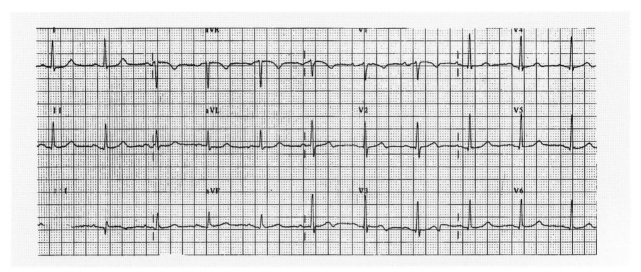

Figure 8.50 *First stage of reperfusion, isoelectric ST segment with decrease in magnitude of the T waves.*

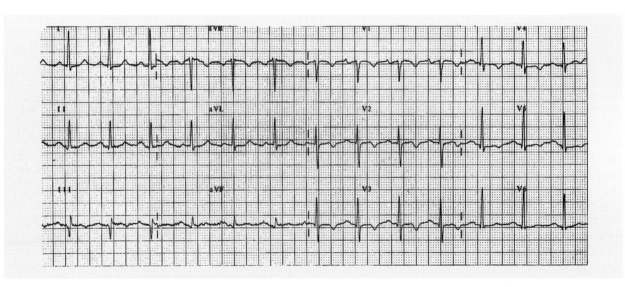

Figure 8.51 *Advanced signs of reperfusion; inverted T waves in the precordial leads.*

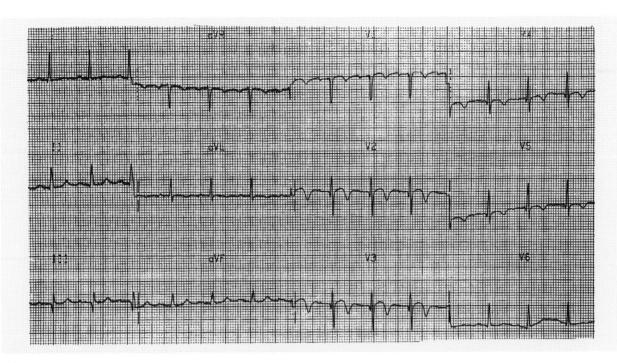

Figure 8.52 *ECG showing subendocardial regional infarcion with a tiny q wave in leads V2–V4, with complete reperfusion, isoelectric ST segment and inverted T waves.*

deeper inverted T waves and the q waves that were more evident, indicating the persistent pattern thereafter.

A coronary angiogram from the patient showed a severe obstruction in the distal left anterior descending coronary artery after the origin of the first diagonal branch (*Fig. 8.53*). The type C artery can be appreciated. Note also the big marginal branch originating from the circumflex artery and supplying the anterolateral wall.

Comments

The patient is protected anatomically (by the marginal branch) and physiologically (Grade 2 ischaemia). The ECGs in *Figs 8.51* and *8.52* depict typical subendocardial infarctions as described in Chapter 4. This is an intermediate pattern between the transmural regional infarction and the regional non-q wave infarction.

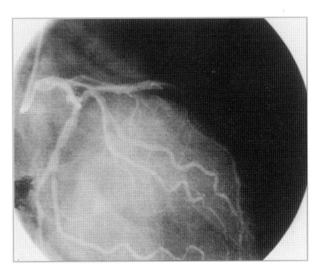

Figure 8.53 *Coronary angiography showing a total obstruction of the 2nd portion of the LAD; the distal portion is perfused by collateral circulation of the big marginal artery.*

CASE 10

Reperfusion QS wave infarction in one anterior lead

A 68-year-old patient with stable angina over the past 3 years arrived at the emergency ward on 6 June 1992 after 5 hours of chest pain. An ECG was recorded at 04.00 (*Fig. 8.54*).

PREINFARCTION STRATIFICATION

The ECG showed preinfarction syndrome (no q-waves) with transmural ischaemia (ST segment elevation) and regional ischaemia (tall and peaked T waves; ischaemia involving anterior precordial leads).

CORONARY ANATOMY

- The culprit artery is the left anterior descending artery (LAD) (maximal changes in leads V2 and V3).
- The level of obstruction is distal to the first diagonal artery (D1) (no ST-segment elevation in lead aVL).
- The dimension of the LAD is type C (ST segment elevation with positive T-waves in lead LIII; reciprocal changes in lead aVL).

MYOCARDIAL ANATOMY

- The core of the myocardial ischaemia, manifested only in lead V2 (see Chapter 2).
- The border zone is large, as demonstrated in leads V3–V6.

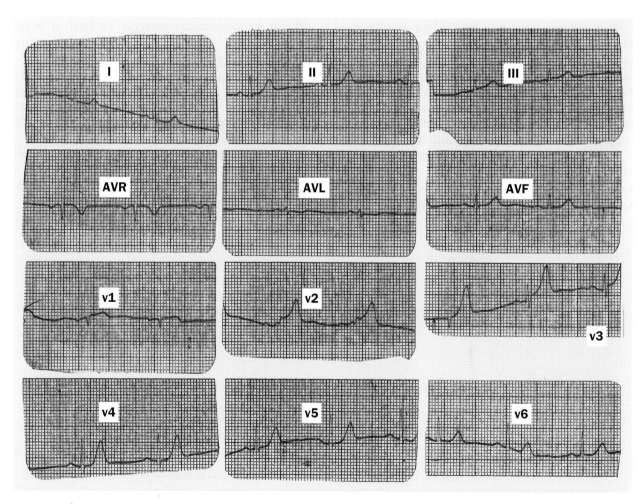

Figure 8.54 *Preinfarction syndrome, transmural regional; ST segment elevation in leads V2–V3 with tall and peaked T waves in all precordial leads.*

- The right side of the septum is supplied both by the conal artery and by the left anterior descending coronary artery, for there is only slight ST segment elevation in lead V1.

PHYSIOLOGY

Ischaemia Grade 3 in only one lead indicates a small unprotected area. Other precordial leads manifest Grade 1 ischaemia, indicating that the myocardium is protected.

The patient received thrombolysis although only one lead was involved. A second ECG was obtained at 06.00 (*Fig. 8.55*). Signs of the initial stage of reperfusion were evident, with 2 mm of ST elevation in leads V2 and V3 and upright T waves, but in lead V2 a reperfusion qS pattern is evident. This is a typical characteristic of regional infarction with reperfusion. The qS wave was 8 mm with a marked notch in the

descending limb. In lead V3 there was a qrS pattern characteristic of subendocardial infarction.

The third ECG (*Fig. 8.56*), obtained at 10.00, showed additional reperfusion with an inverted T wave in all precordial leads.

The fourth ECG (*Fig. 8.57*), obtained 2 days later, showed complete reperfusion with deep, inverted T waves in all precordial leads and an isoelectric ST segment in leads V4–V6. There was persistent ST segment elevation in lead V2.

Echocardiography (*Fig. 8.58*), performed on the third day, showed that the apex and the inferior and anterior walls are akinetic. The cardiac dimensions are normal.

Coronary angiography (*Fig. 8.59*) showed critical thrombotic obstruction in LAD, distal to D1. The LAD wraps the apex and a large marginal supplies the anterolateral wall.

Comments
This interesting case shows a very small zone that is

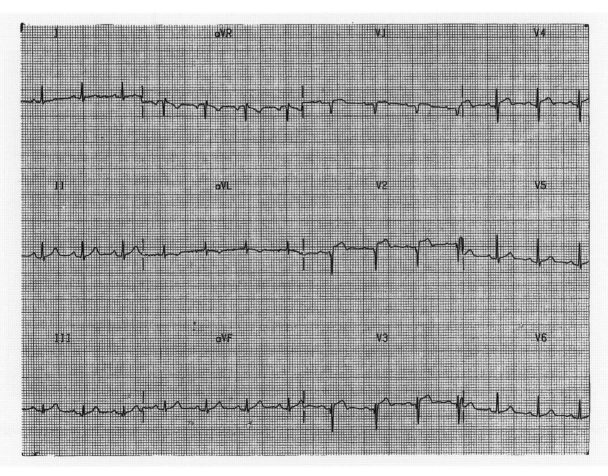

Figure 8.55 *Incomplete first stage of reperfusion; q-wave infarction. ST segment elevation in leads V2–V3 with reduced magnitude of the T waves in all precordial leads.*

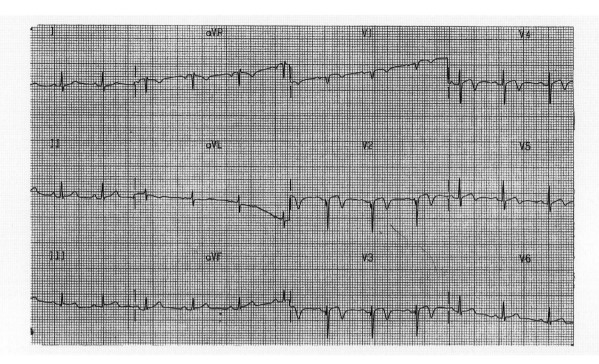

Figure 8.56 *ECG showing 2nd stage of reperfusion in leads V2–V5.*

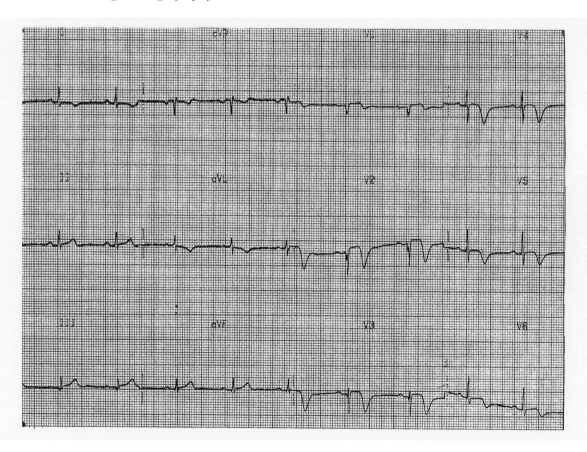

Figure 8.57 *Reperfusion, q-wave infarcion; qs with a 'notch wave' in lead V2; isoelectric ST segment and inverted T waves in all precordial leads.*

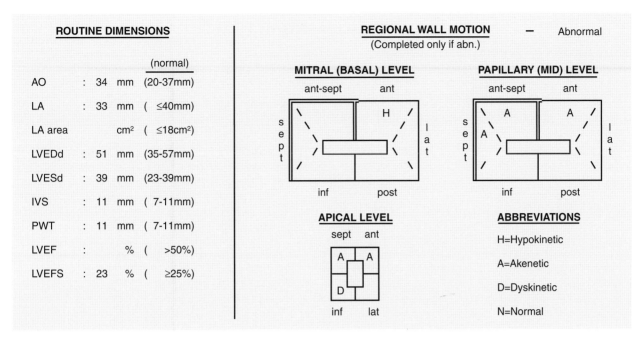

ROUTINE DIMENSIONS			
			(normal)
AO	: 34	mm	(20-37mm)
LA	: 33	mm	(≤40mm)
LA area		cm²	(≤18cm²)
LVEDd	: 51	mm	(35-57mm)
LVESd	: 39	mm	(23-39mm)
IVS	: 11	mm	(7-11mm)
PWT	: 11	mm	(7-11mm)
LVEF	:	%	(>50%)
LVEFS	: 23	%	(≥25%)

REGIONAL WALL MOTION — Abnormal
(Completed only if abn.)

MITRAL (BASAL) LEVEL

PAPILLARY (MID) LEVEL

APICAL LEVEL

ABBREVIATIONS

H=Hypokinetic

A=Akenetic

D=Dyskinetic

N=Normal

Figure 8.58 *Echocardiogram showing akinesia in the anteroseptal and anterior wall, in the apical and upper surrounding area.*

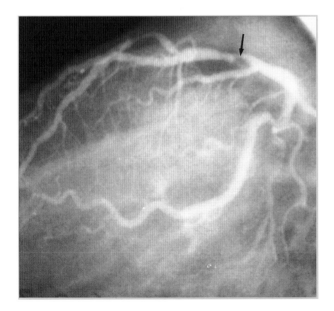

Figure 8.59 *Coronary angiography showing a thrombotic obstruction of the LAD (arrow) with reperfusion TIMI 3. Note the big marginal branch supplying the anterolateral wall.*

not protected surrounded by a well-protected area. In lead V2 there is a transmural qS transmural infarction, in V3 there is a qrS subendocardial infarction, and in leads V4 and V5 there is non-q wave infarction. This can be viewed as a gradient in severity of injury.

CASE 11

More advanced reperfusion QS wave infarction

A 58-year-old patient was admitted to the coronary care unit after 3½ hours of chest pain on 6 August 1992 at 11.00. An ECG was recorded on admission (*Fig. 8.60*).

PREINFARCTION STRATIFICATION

The ECG showed preinfarction syndrome (no Q waves); the qS in lead V2 is probably the result of an unknown, old anteroseptal wall myocardial infarction, transmural ischaemia (ST segment elevation), and regional ischaemia (positive T waves; anterior wall, precordial leads from leads V2–V5).

CORONARY ANATOMY

- The culprit artery is the left anterior descending artery (LAD), with maximal changes in leads V2 and V3.
- The level of obstruction is proximal to the first diagonal artery (D1) (ST segment elevation and positive T-waves in lead aVL).
- The dimension of the LAD is type B (ST segment depression and negative T-waves in lead LIII; the ST segment elevation and T wave in lead aVL are higher than ST segment elevation and T wave in lead LI.

MYOCARDIAL ANATOMY

- The core of the myocardial ischaemia is large (seen in leads V2–V6).
- The border zone is not seen; most probably, marginal arteries do not supply the anterolateral

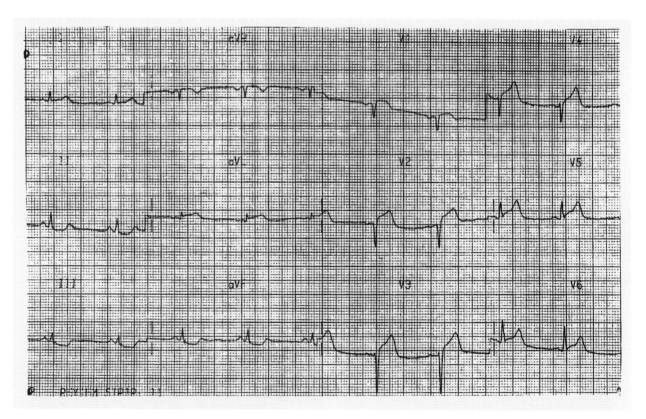

Figure 8.60 *Preinfarction syndrome, transmural regional anterior wall; the poor progression of the r waves in leads V2–V4 represent most probably an old anteroseptal wall infarction. Note, the ST segment elevation with positve T waves in leads LI and aVL and non-q waves in these leads, indicating a new obstruction as well as the ST segment elevation and positive T waves in leads V5–V6.*

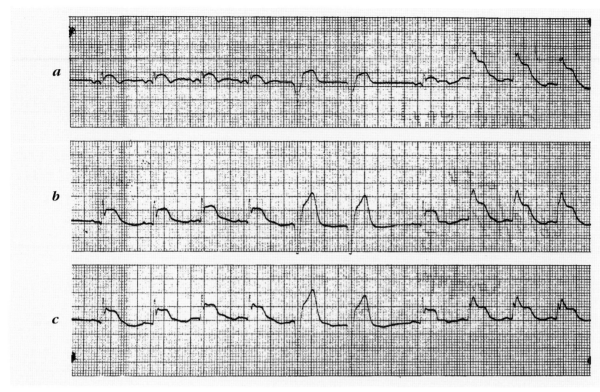

Figure 8.61 *ECG showing three different complications of reperfusion. (a) Reperfusion injury: the first 4 sinus beats are simultaneous recording of V1–V2–V3 showing re-elevation of ST segments and R waves (fading the q waves) but without changes in the magnitude of the T waves. The last 3 sinus beats are simultaneous recording of V4–V5–V6, showing re-elevation of ST segments with increase in the magnitude of the R wave. No change in the magnitude of the T waves. (b) Early reperfusion RBBB: the first 4 beats in lead V1 show a RBBB pattern. (c) Reperfusion arrhythmias: accelerated idioventricular rhythm; beats 5–6 are ventricular rhythm with a frequency of 75 bpm.*

wall and the absence of the border zone indicates that the LAD supplies the anterolateral wall.

• The right side of the septum is supplied by the LAD because of the 2 mm ST segment elevation in lead V1 (an attenuation phenomenon between lead V1 and leads V5–V6).

PHYSIOLOGY

Ischaemia Grade 2 with tall, peaked T-waves indicates a moderately protected myocardium.

The ECG was recorded 40 minutes after commencement of thrombolytic therapy. The first seven beats of the subsequent ECG (*Fig. 8.61*) show leads V1–V3 and the last three beats show leads V5 and V6. There was re-elevation of the ST segment and an increase in the amplitude of the R wave but not of the T wave. The fifth and sixth beats are accelerated idioventricular rhythms. (There are two manifestations of reperfusion—re-elevation of the ST segment without re-elevation of the T wave, which is type 1 re-ischaemia related to myocardial injury, as opposed to a tall, peaked T wave and reperfusion arrhythmias.)

The third ECG (*Fig. 8.62*) was obtained 1 hour after thrombolytic therapy. This ECG showed marked signs of reperfusion with a marked resolution of the ST segment elevation. However, right bundle branch block with left anterior hemiblock has developed. The second vector of the right bundle branch block is wide (120 msec), as seen in leads aVR and L2. (This is reperfusion right bundle branch block as described in Chapter 7.)

Two days later, an ECG (*Fig. 8.63*) showed advanced stages of reperfusion with inverted T waves from leads V1–V6 and in leads L1 and aVL. Note that leads V2–V4 maintained a small r wave, but the q waves are localized to leads V5 and aVL.

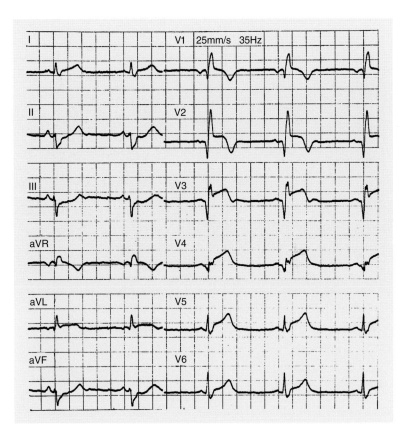

Figure 8.62 *ECG showing complete reperfusion; RBBB with left axis deviation.*

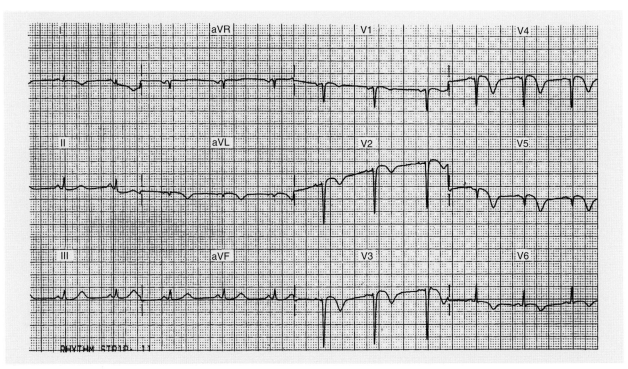

Figure 8.63 *ECG showing extensive reperfusion, q-wave-infarction involving all the precordial leads as well as LI and aVL. Note the pronounced inverted T waves in leads V4–V6 with isoelectric ST segment in leads V2–V3; slight elevation of the ST segment and moderate depth of the T waves.*

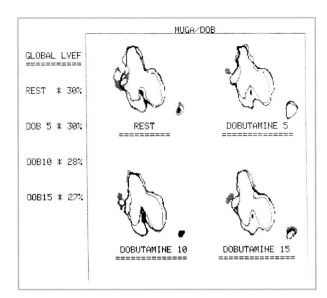

Figure 8.64 *MUGA study with an increasing dose of dopamine; no change in ventricular contraction.*

This is a type of infarction with good reperfusion. It is difficult to categorize this infarction as q wave or non-q wave This case is a more extensive infarction than case 10.

On 15 August 1992, a multiple-gated acquisition scan of the heart (*Fig. 8.64*) in the left anterior oblique view depicted regional abnormality of wall motion at rest with a global ejection fraction of 30 per cent. When dobutamine was administered, there was no improvement in contraction. However, 2 months later, this test was repeated; this time there was improved contraction, indicating that the heart had been stunned during the initial test.

CASE 12

Early angioplasty and reperfusion QS-wave infarction

A 50-year-old man arrived at the hospital on 30 December 1997 because of recent unstable angina. In the emergency room, he developed severe chest pain and was treated for ventricular fibrillation. An ECG was obtained immediately after resuscitation at 10.00 (*Fig. 8.65*). Preinfarction syndrome involving all the precordial leads was evident, with ST segment elevation and tall, peaked T waves.

PREINFARCTION STRATIFICATION

The ECG showed preinfarction syndrome. The tiny q waves do not indicate necrosis; in this case the early q waves were caused by depression in the conduction of the Purkinje fibers in the ischaemic area. There is transmural ischaemia (ST segment elevation), regional ischaemia (tall and peaked T waves), and anterior wall ischaemia (precordial leads).

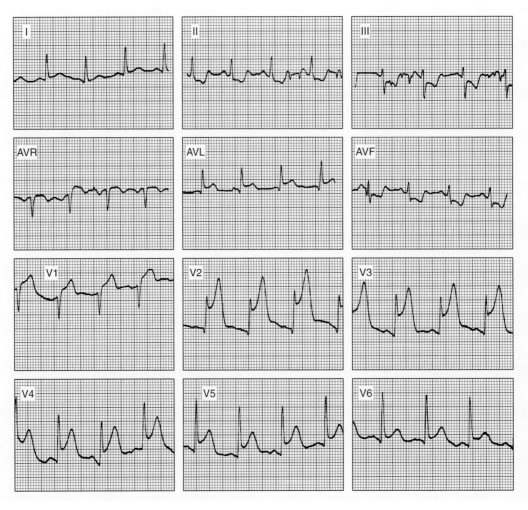

Figure 8.65 *Preinfarction syndrome, transmural regional; extensive, anterior wall.*

CORONARY ANATOMY

- The culprit artery is the left anterior descending artery, with maximal changes in leads V2–V3.
- The level of obstruction is proximal to the first diagonal artery (D1) (ST segment elevation in lead aVL).
- The dimension of LAD is type B (ST segment depression and negative T waves in lead LIII); the ST–T changes in lead aVL are greater than those in lead LI.

MYOCARDIAL ANATOMY

- The core of myocardial ischaemia is very extensive (as seen in leads V2–V6).
- The border zone is not seen (there is no marginal artery supply of the anterolateral wall).
- The right side of the septum is involved (lead V1 showed ST segment elevation with positive T waves; there is an attenuation phenomenon between lead V1 and leads V5–V6).

PHYSIOLOGY

There is ischaemia Grade 3 in leads V2–V4 and ischaemia Grade 2 in leads V5 and V6. The core is thus unprotected.

The patient was transferred to the catheterization laboratory at 11.45. The catheter study (*Fig. 8.66*) showed a very proximal obstruction of the LAD. After angioplasty and stent implantation, the artery remained patent. An ECG was obtained immediately after reperfusion (*Fig. 8.67*). A qS wave was seen in leads V2 and V3 and signs of stage 2 of myocardial reperfusion were evident (ST elevation and positive T1 with inverted T2 in leads V2 and V3). The next day, an ECG (*Fig. 8.68*) depicted complete reperfusion in a manner typical for qS infarc-

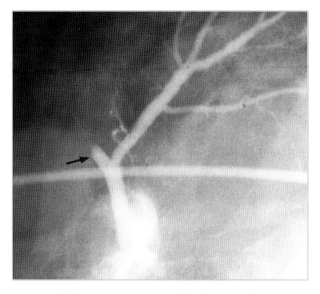

Figure 8.66 *Coronary angiography showing a total obstruction of the intial portion of the left anterior descending artery.*

tion—qS in lead V2 and a qrS pattern in lead V3. Deep inverted T waves with slight ST elevation were seen in leads V2 and V3. Sestamibi scintigraphic images (*Fig. 8.69*) showed good left ventricular contraction with a small defect in the anteroapical aspect. This pattern is typical for reperfusion QS wave infarctions.

Comments

Patients who present with ischaemia Grade 3 must be treated promptly because the window of opportunity is brief. This is in contrast to patients with lesser degrees of ischaemia, as discussed in Chapter 4. This patient was fortunate to be treated on the spot for what was a potentially lethal infarction. It is also important to stress that patients with ischaemia Grade 3 often manifest transient q waves early. These are manifestations of conduction defects and do not denote a process of necrosis.

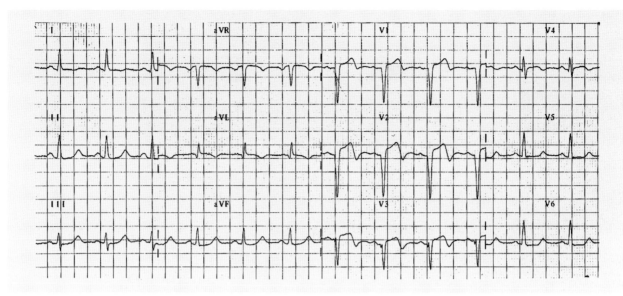

Figure 8.67 *ECG recorded immediately after angioplasty; 2nd stage of reperfusion; inverted T_2 waves in leads V2–V3, with elevation of T_1 waves and ST segment and reperfusion QS in V2–V3.*

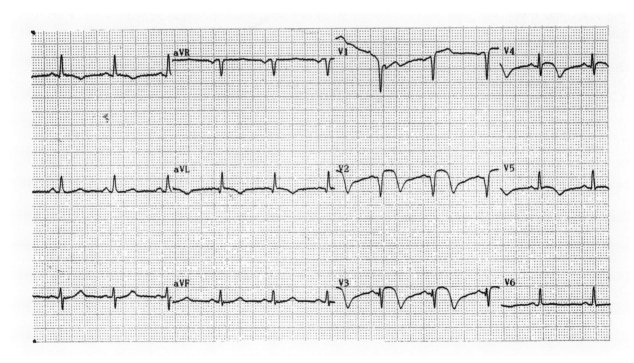

Figure 8.68 *Reperfusion, q-wave infarction; qs in lead V2 (7 mm); deep inverted T waves in leads V2–V5 and ST segment elevation in leads V2–V3.*

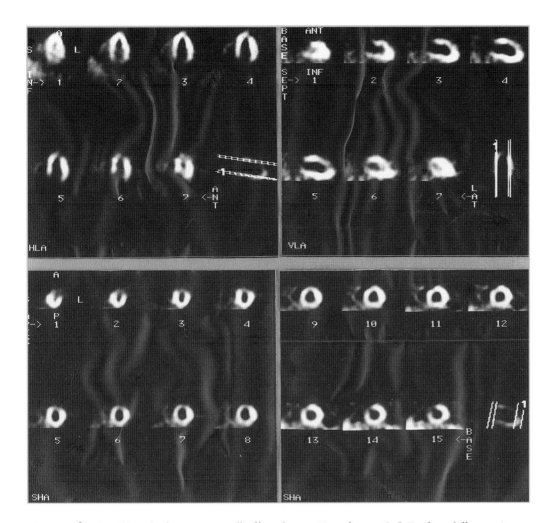

Figure 8.69 *SPECT study showing a small affected area. Note, frames 5–6–7– four different views.*

CASE 13

Extensive Q-wave infarction

A 47-year-old man with a history of smoking and hypercholesterolaemia was admitted to the emergency ward 90 minutes after the onset of chest pain. An ECG (*Fig. 8.70*) was obtained on admission (25 December 1997 at 09.00).

PREINFARCTION STRATIFICATION

The ECG showed preinfarction syndrome (the tiny q waves seen in leads V2 and V3 in this case are due to a depression in the conduction of the Purkinje fibers in the ischaemic area). There was transmural ischaemia (ST segment elevation), regional ischaemia (tall and peaked T waves), and anterior wall ischaemia (involvement of precordial leads).

CORONARY ANATOMY

- The culprit artery is the left anterior descending artery (LAD), with maximal changes in leads V2 and V3.
- The level of the obstruction is probably proximal (there is ST elevation in lead aVL but no positive T waves—these are undiagnosable findings).
- The dimension of the LAD is suspected type C (there is attenuation of the ischaemic manifestations between leads aVL and LIII).

MYOCARDIAL ANATOMY

- The core of the myocardial ischaemia is very extensive (see in leads V2–V5).
- The border zone is not seen.
- The right side of the septum is involved (ST segment elevation with positive T waves in lead V1; attenuation phenomenon between the two opposite ischaemic areas represented by lead V1 and leads V5 and V6).

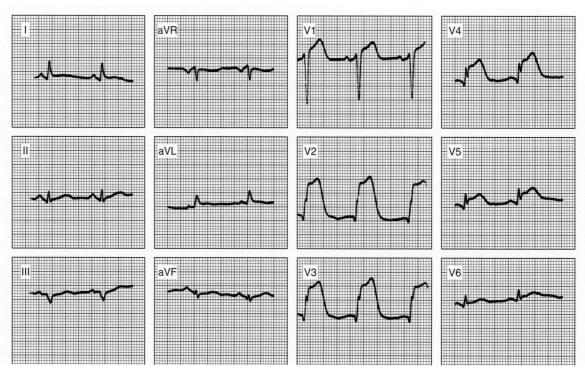

Figure 8.70 *Preinfarction syndrome, transmural regional with a tiny q-wave in leads V2–V3.*

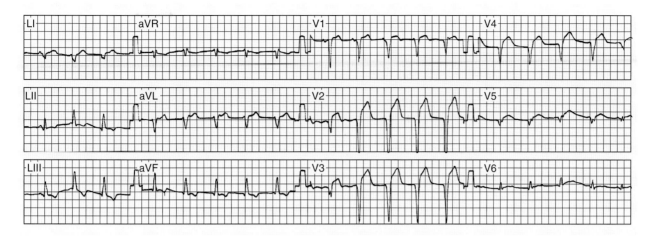

Figure 8.71 *ECG showing an accelerated idioventricular rhythm with LBBB like pattern and extreme right axis deviation.*

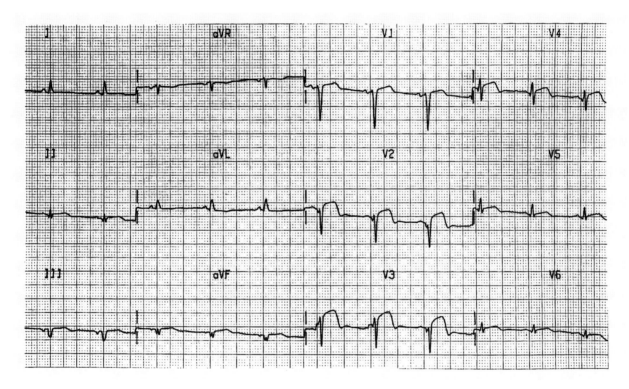

Figure 8.72 *ECG showing 2nd stage of reperfusion (incomplete); commencement of T_2 wave inversion with T_1 wave elevation as well as ST segments in leads V2–V5.*

PHYSIOLOGY

Ischaemia Grade 3 denotes an unprotected myocardium.

The patient received thrombolytic therapy along with aspirin and heparin. Twenty minutes after treatment an ECG (*Fig. 8.71*) showed accelerated idioventricular rhythm with a left bundle branch block-like pattern and extreme right axis deviation, suggesting that the focus is located in the right side of the septum. The first beat in leads V1–V3 was a sinus conducted beat, indicating a very advanced degree of reperfusion.

Reperfusion QS waves developed in lead V2 and

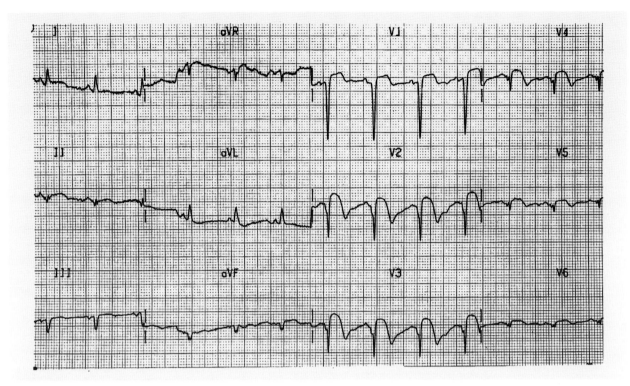

Figure 8.73 *ECG showing reperfusion Q-wave infarction: qs in leads V2–V4 with a descending 'notch wave'; inverted T waves in precordial leads with ST segment elevation in leads V2–V6.*

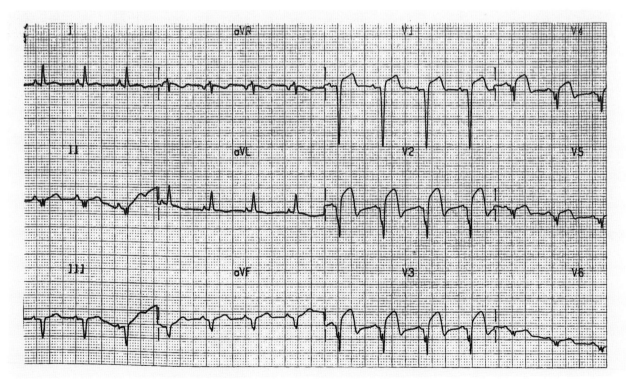

Figure 8.74 *Re-elevation of ST segments in leads V2–V5 with decrease in the depth of the T waves (no anginal pain).*

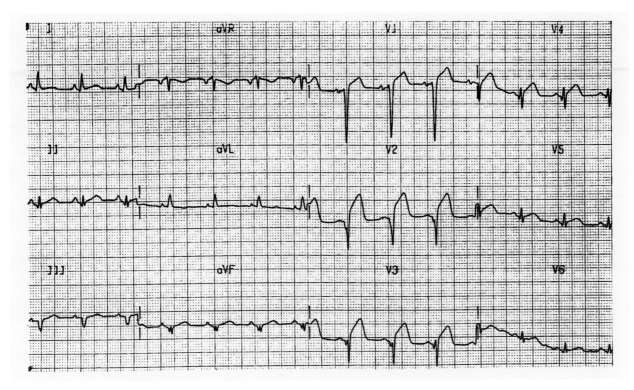

Figure 8.75 *ECG showing the predicted evolution of ST–T changes; the T waves become positive.*

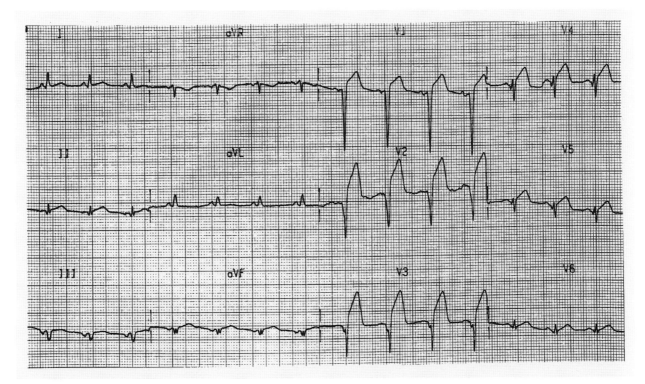

Figure 8.76 *ST–T changes evolving to their maximal dimension. Note, the pronounced ST segment elevation and positive T waves (no anginal pain); (see the difference with the ischaemic second peak of the ST–T in Case 2, Figs 4, 5 and 6).*

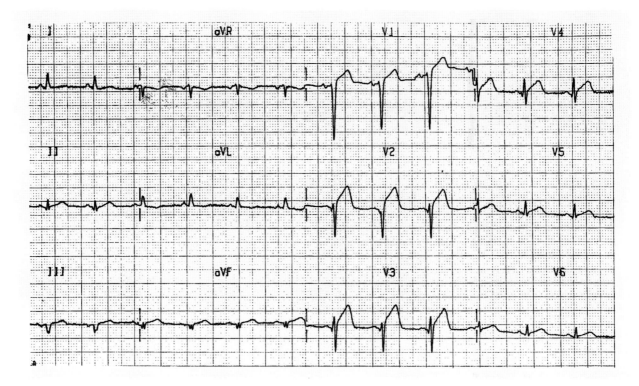

Figure 8.77 *ECG showing the progressive reduction in the magnitude of the ST–T.*

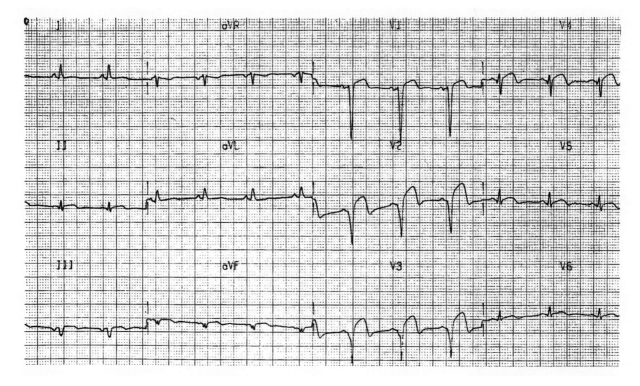

Figure 8.78 *ECG showing a progressive inversion of T_2 waves.*

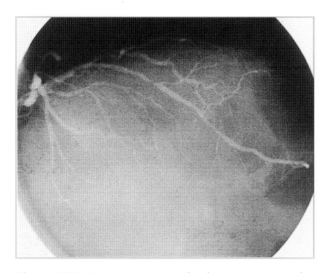

Figure 8.79 *Coronary angiography showing a proximal LAD obstruction with TIMI 2.*

inverted T2 in the same lead. An ECG obtained later that day (*Fig. 8.72*) showed a sinus rhythm with a similar stage of reperfusion. The next ECG (*Fig. 8.73*) showed more advanced stages of reperfusion, with inverted T waves, ST elevation in leads V2–V6, and reperfusion qS infarction waves.

An ECG obtained on 26 December (*Fig. 8.74*) showed that the ST segments are higher than they had been the previous day and that the T wave has become less inverted. An ECG 2 days later (*Fig. 8.75*) shows that the T waves are upright and that the ST is still higher. On 30 December very tall T waves with ST segment elevation were noted (*Fig. 8.76*). The next day, the ECG showed partial resolution of these changes (*Fig. 8.77*). One day later, T2 has become inverted (*Fig. 8.78*). Throughout this period, the patient was completely asymptomatic.

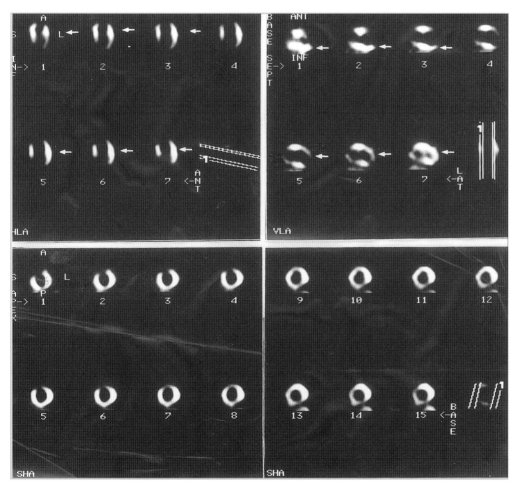

Figure 8.80 *SPECT study showing through the four views an extensive anteroseptal and anterior wall infarction.*

Coronary angiography (*Fig. 8.79*) was performed on 2 January 1998. A thrombotic occlusion of the proximal LAD is noted with another narrowing in the distal segment. Note that the artery extends beyond the apex and that the small circumflex artery does not supply the anterolateral wall. Sestamibi scintigraphy (*Fig. 8.80*) on 28 December 1997 revealed a large perfusion defect involving the anterior, anterolateral, apical and inferior walls.

Comments

This patient had severe anatomical and physiological parameters. After 3 hours, the prognosis is severe even if reperfusion is instituted. This patient was treated within 90 minutes of onset of pain. The second ECG showed signs of reperfusion with a resolution of ST segment elevation. The subsequent second peak of ST segment elevation could be predicted by the initial pattern of reperfusion. We think that it does not denote re-ischaemia, but rather reflects myocardial expansion. In this case, despite the early reperfusion, the patient still had a very large perfusion defect.

CASE 14

Non-reperfusion Q wave infarction

A 40-year-old man had suffered an inferior myocardial infarct 1 year ago. He had undergone angioplasty of the right coronary artery. The patient woke from sleep on 20 November 1992 with severe anginal pain. He arrived at 05.00 in the coronary care unit after four hours of pain. An ECG was recorded on arrival (*Fig. 8.81*).

PREINFARCTION STRATIFICATION

The ECG showed preinfarction syndrome (no q waves), transmural ischaemia (ST elevation), regional ischaemia (tall peaked T waves), and anterior wall ischaemia (visible in the precordial leads).

CORONARY ANATOMY

- The culprit artery is the left anterior descending artery (LAD), with maximal changes in leads V2, V3, and V4.
- The level of obstruction is proximal to the first diagonal artery (D1) (ST elevation and positive T wave in lead aVL).
- The dimension of the artery is type C (wrapping the apex) (the ST–T changes in lead I are greater than those in lead aVL; there is ST depression in lead LIII with positive T waves; there is attenuation between leads aVL and LIII).

MYOCARDIAL ANATOMY

- The core of myocardial ischaemia is very extensive (leads V2–V5).

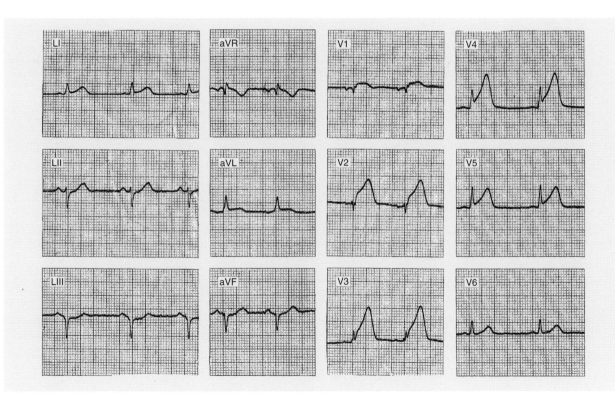

Figure 8.81 *Preinfarction syndromes, transmural regional anterior wall.*

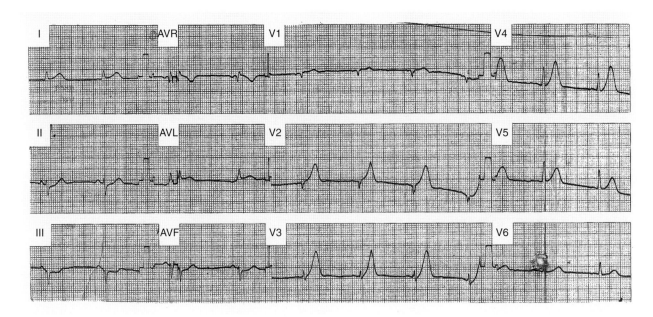

Figure 8.82 *First stage of reperfusion; moderate ST segment elevation with positive T waves in the precordial leads.*

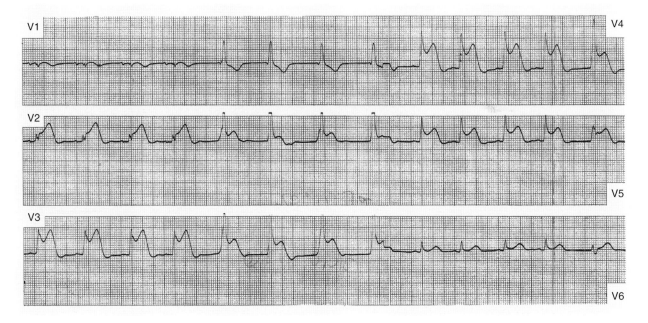

Figure 8.83 *Two complications of reperfusion; the first 7 beats were simultaneously recorded in leads V1–V2–V3; the last 5 beats were simultaneously recorded in leads V4–V5–V6. The sinus beat, the first 4 beats and the last 9–12 beats show a re-elevation of the ST segment and the T waves (phasic flow variation); the 5–8 beats as well as the last beat, are accelerated idioventricular rhythm (AIVR).*

- There is no border zone.
- The right side of the septum is involved (ST elevation with positive T wave—attenuation between leads V1 and V6).

PHYSIOLOGY

There is Grade 2 ischaemia with deformation of the S wave in lead V3.

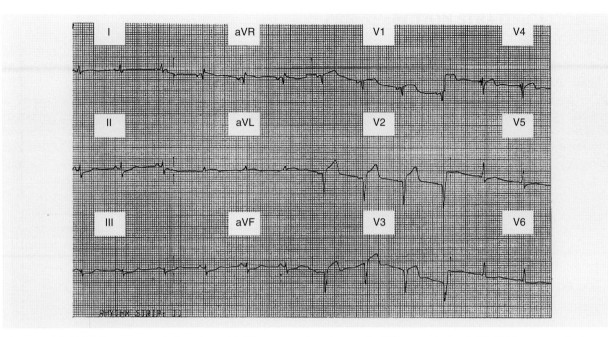

Figure 8.84 *ECG showing a qs infarction with ST segment elevation and tall T waves in leads V2–V3 (non-reperfusion-q-wave-infarction).*

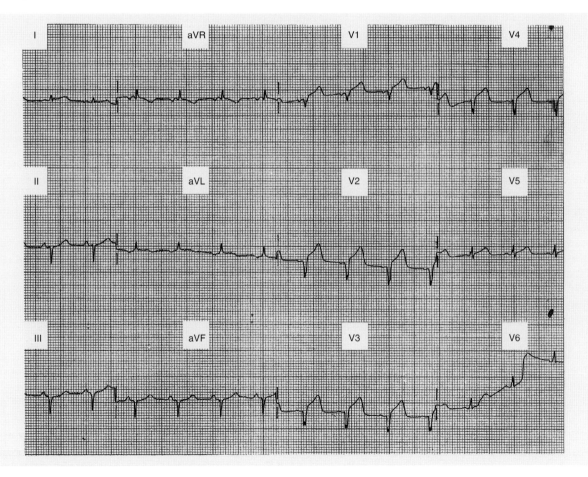

Figure 8.85 *Non-reperfused Q-wave infarction.*

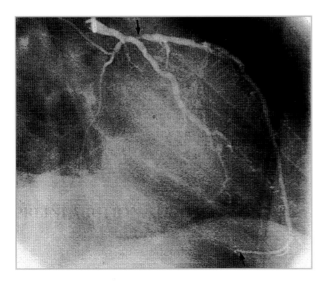

Figure 8.86 *Coronary angiography showing a very high LAD obstruction.*

Figure 8.87 *MUGA study with progressive doses of dopamine showing no improvement in the myocardial function; severe myocardial dysfunction.*

The patient received aspirin (350 mg) and heparin 5000 U.

An ECG at 05.30 (*Fig. 8.82*) showed signs of epicardial reperfusion, a slight decrease in the magnitude of the T wave, no change in the QRS complex, but a significant reduction of the ST segment. There were no changes in the standard leads, probably representing non-reperfusion of the D1 area (ST elevation in leads LI and aVL and ST depression in lead LIII). Despite signs of reperfusion, the patient received thrombolytic treatment.

An ECG obtained at 07.30 (*Fig. 8.83*) is shown—the first four beats are sinus rhythm recorded simultaneously in V1 to V3; the beats show a re-elevation of ST segments and increasing magnitude of T waves and R waves (phasic flow variation of reperfusion ischaemia) (see Chapter 3). The next four beats are accelerated idioventricular rhythm recorded in V2–V3. Note the pattern of RBBB-like, with a frequency of 75 bpm. The beats 9 to 12 are also sinus rhythm recorded simultaneously in V4–V5–V6. Note, that the grade of ischaemia (grade 3) is higher in these leads than in the pre-treated patient.

The last beat is a ventricular escape (see Chapter 6, Reperfusion extrasystoles). This strip shows two reperfusion phenomena:

- A marked increase of ST segment elevation and T waves in the precordial leads.
- Accelerated idioventricular rhythm.

The origin of the ventricular rhythm is located in the upper part (all beats are positive) of the left ventricle, RBBB-like pattern (positive R wave from leads V1–V5).

Two days later, an ECG (*Fig. 8.84*) showed signs of non-reperfusion q wave infarction. There was significant ST elevation in leads V2 and V3, with tall T waves.

Nine days later, an ECG (*Fig. 8.85*) still showed non-reperfusion q wave infarction.

Coronary angiography was performed on 26 November 1992 (*Fig. 8.86*). It showed thrombotic obstruction in the proximal part of the LAD. The LAD is type C, wrapping the apex. No second marginal artery was seen.

Multiple gated acquisition scan of the heart with dopamine test (*Fig. 8.87*) showed a 30% ejection fraction at rest. Increased dose of dopamine produced no changes on the contraction, indicating severe damage to the myocardium.

Comments

This patient was admitted with a very extensive and moderately protected preinfarction syndrome of the anterior wall. Administration of heparin and aspirin probably reduced the thrombus and allowed the typical changes of regional subendocardial preinfarction. The thrombolysis produced a complicated reperfusion.

CASE 15

Severe hypertension induced left ventricle hypertrophy

A 73-year-old man with severe systemic hypertension was admitted to the emergency room after 4 hours of severe pain. The first ECG was recorded at 14.00 on 17 February 1998 (*Fig. 8.88*). It showed severe left ventricular hypertrophy with no progression of the R wave from lead V1 to lead V3.

Preinfarction stratification

The ECG is considered to show the preinfarction syndrome anterior wall in the presence of left ventricular hypertrophy.

CORONARY ANATOMY

• The culprit artery is the left anterior descending artery (LAD), with maximal changes in leads V1 and V3.
• The level of obstruction is proximal to the first diagonal artery (D1) (ST elevation and positive T waves in lead aVL).

• The dimension of the LAD is type B (ST depression and negative T waves in lead LIII, ST–T changes in lead aVL greater than those in lead LI).

MYOCARDIAL ANATOMY

• The ST segment elevation involves leads from V2 to V5, therefore the core of myocardial ischaemia is very large.
• No ST segment elevation in lead V6 indicates that the border zone is very small.
• There is suspected right ventricular involvement (though this pattern also appears in left ventricular hypertrophy). The ST segment elevation and upright T wave in lead V1 can be induced by acute ischaemia of the right side of the septum or by systolic overloading in severe left ventricular hypertrophy.

Physiology

There is Grade 2 ischaemia (as shown in leads V2–V5 with tall peaked T waves), and the myocardium is moderately protected.

The patient was treated by thrombolytic therapy. Two hours later there were no signs of reperfusion

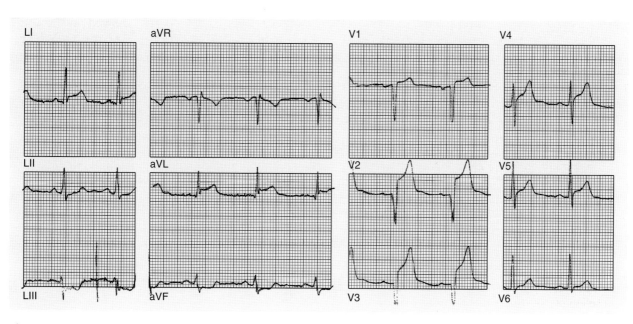

Figure 8.88 *ECG showing preinfarction syndrome, transmural regional anterior wall.*

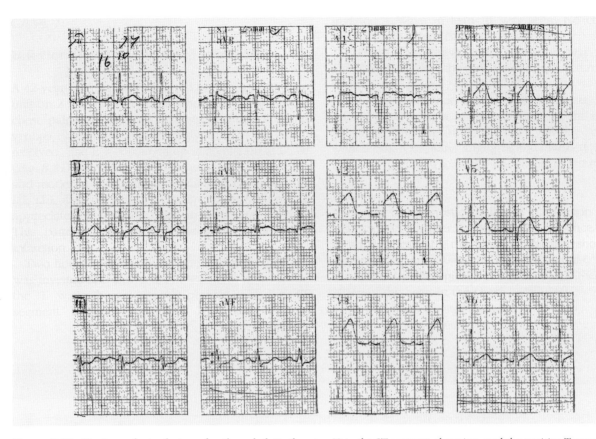

Figure 8.89 *No signs of reperfusion after thrombolytic therapy. Note the ST segment elevation and the positive T waves.*

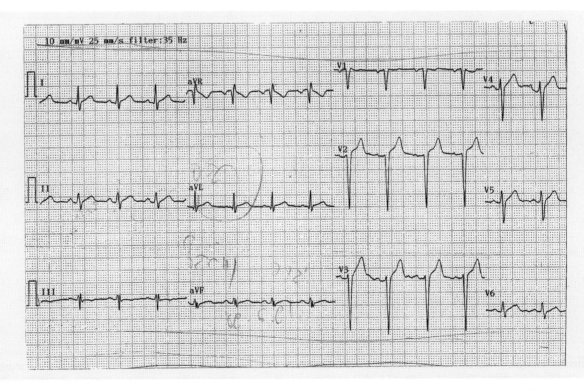

Figure 8.90 *ST segment elevation with positive T waves in the precordial leads and ST segment elevation with positive T waves in aVL and LI three hours after thrombolytic therapy.*

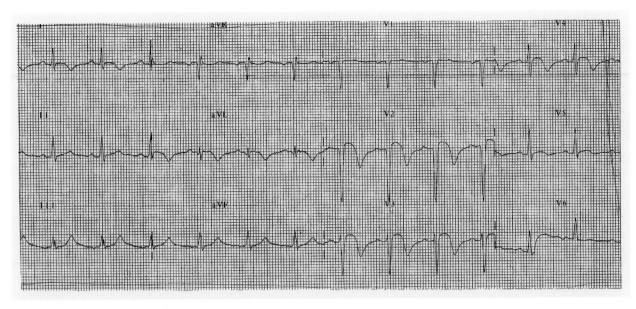

Figure 8.91 *ECG recorded just before coronary angiography was performed. Note the signs of complete reperfusion: inverted T waves in leads V2–V3 with a very slight ST segment elevation.*

(*Fig. 8.89*). At 17.00 the patient was taken for rescue percutaneous transluminal coronary angioplasty. Just before the procedure, the ECG showed inverted T waves and ST segment depression, signs of complete reperfusion (*Fig. 8.90*). The coronary angiography, 15 minutes later, showed thrombotic obstruction with TIMI 3 flow (*Fig. 8.91*).

The echocardiogram obtained on the third day showed extensive akinesia in the apical and middle parts of the anterior septal wall.

Comments

This patient was admitted after 4 hours of pain with extensive Grade 2 ischaemia. Signs of reperfusion could not be detected 2.5 hours after thrombolysis. However, the ECG showed spontaneous complete reperfusion of the anterior wall, confirmed by TIMI 3 coronary flow. Despite 7 hours of obstruction, complete reperfusion was observed.

CASE 16

Reperfusion right bundle branch block

A 73-year-old man was admitted to the coronary care unit after 3 hours of pain on 27 June 1997 at 12.00.

Preinfarction stratification

The first ECG showed preinfarction syndrome; the small q wave in lead V2 was due to extreme left anterior hemiblock (*Fig. 8.92*).

CORONARY ANATOMY

- The culprit artery is the left anterior descending artery, with maximal changes in leads V2 and V3.
- The level of obstruction is proximal to the first diagonal artery (D1) (ST elevation and positive T waves in lead aVL).
- The dimension of the LAD is type C (attenuated ST segment elevation and the dimension of the T waves in aVL as well as ST segment depression and T wave in lead LIII).

MYOCARDIAL ANATOMY

- The core of the myocardial ischaemia is very small (leads V2 and V3).
- The border zone is large. Grade 1 ischaemia is extended from lead V3 to V6, indicating a well protected area.
- There is right ventricular involvement (ST elevation in lead V1).

PHYSIOLOGY

There is ischaemia Grade 2 (seen in lead V2), and ischaemia Grade 1 (seen in leads V3–V6). The myocardium is well protected, probably because of a large second marginal artery.

The patient was treated with thrombolysis and heparin. After 40 minutes, re-ischaemia appeared, with right bundle branch block and a very wide left anterior hemiblock (*Fig. 8.93*). The second vector of the right bundle branch block is 160 msec wide. (This special pattern was discussed in Chapter 7; it is a consequence of the metabolic effect of the very early reperfusion on the conduction system; note that the right side of the septum was involved indicated by ST segment elevation and positive T wave in V1.)

An ECG recorded at 16.00 showed very advanced stages of reperfusion (*Fig. 8.94*). The wide bundle branch block progressively disappeared. Two days later an ECG showed a reperfusion q wave infarction on lead V2 and non-q wave reperfusion in leads V3–V6 (*Fig. 8.95*).

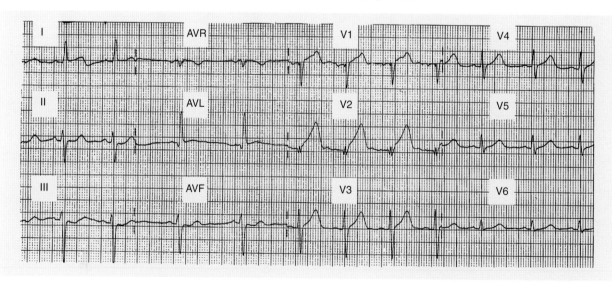

Figure 8.92 *Preinfarcton syndrome, transmural regional anterior wall. Note the ST segment elevation in lead V1 and the 'attenuation phenomenon' between aVL-aVF.*

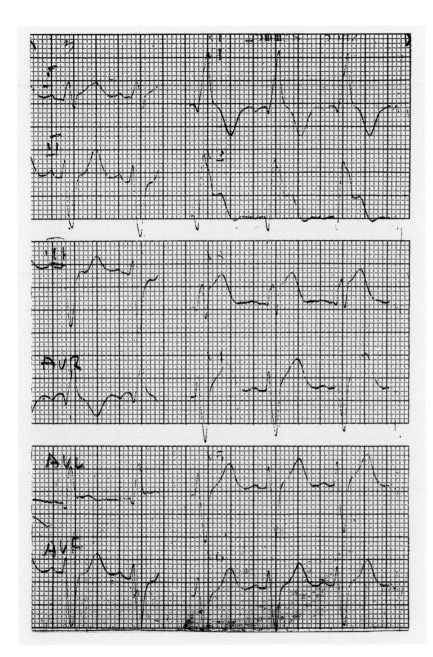

Figure 8.93 *ECG showing complete reperfusion; RBBB with LAHB.*

Comments

This patient presented with a highly protected myocardium. Thrombolysis caused two complications of reperfusion—re-ischaemic phenomenon and reperfusion right bundle branch block. Despite these complications, the patient developed a one-lead reperfusion Q wave and a reperfusion non-Q wave infarction in the other leads.

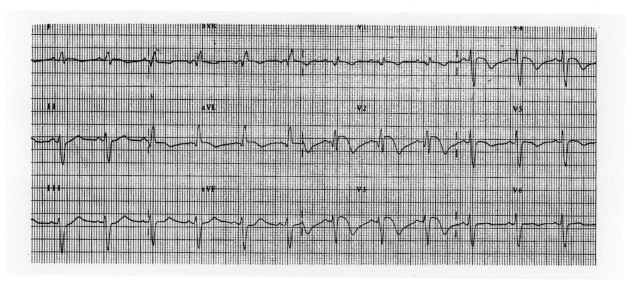

Figure 8.94 *ECG showing more advanced signs of reperfusion and commencement of the complete RBBB disappearance.*

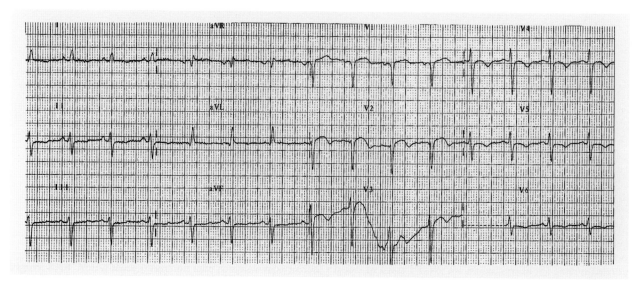

Figure 8.95 *ECG showing Q-wave reperfusion in lead V2 without bundle branch block.*

Index